OVERCOMING SLEEP DISORDERS
Naturally

LAUREL VUKOVIC, M.S.W.

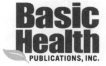

Basic Health
PUBLICATIONS, INC.

The information contained in this book is based upon the research and personal and professional experiences of the author. It is not intended as a substitute for consulting with your physician or other healthcare provider. Any attempt to diagnose and treat an illness should be done under the direction of a healthcare professional.

The publisher does not advocate the use of any particular healthcare protocol but believes the information in this book should be available to the public. The publisher and author are not responsible for any adverse effects or consequences resulting from the use of the suggestions, preparations, or procedures discussed in this book. Should the reader have any questions concerning the appropriateness of any procedures or preparation mentioned, the author and the publisher strongly suggest consulting a professional healthcare advisor.

Basic Health Publications, Inc.
28812 Top of the World Drive
Laguna Beach, CA 92651
949-715-7327

Library of Congress Cataloging-in-Publication Data
Vukovic, Laurel.
  Overcoming sleep disorders naturally / Laurel Vukovic.
     p. cm.
  Includes bibliographical references and index.
  ISBN-13: 978-1-59120-096-3
  1. Sleep—Popular works. 2. Insomnia—Popular works. I. Title.

  RA786.V85   2004
  616.8'498—dc22
                                            2005007431

Editor: Kate Johnson
Typesetting/Book design: Gary A. Rosenberg
Cover design: Mike Stromberg

Printed in the United States of America

10   9   8   7   6   5   4   3   2   1

Contents

Introduction

If you've picked up this book, chances are you have trouble sleeping. Perhaps you have difficulty falling asleep. Or, you might fall asleep easily but then awaken during the night and find it impossible to get back to sleep. You might even think you're sleeping a sufficient number of hours but still wake up tired and groggy in the morning. Any of these situations indicates that you may have a sleep disorder. The most familiar sleep disorder, of course, is insomnia.

If you do have trouble sleeping, you're certainly not alone. More than one third of adults in the United States experience occasional insomnia and at least one out of ten American adults suffers from chronic insomnia. As you know if you've suffered even one night of insomnia, the consequences of sleep impairment or deprivation also affect your waking hours. A lack of restful sleep causes mood disturbances, impairs mental and physical performance, wears down the immune system, and ages you more quickly. It's all too easy for a sleep disturbance to become a recurring problem. Fortunately, there are many things you can do to break this exhausting cycle.

In this book, you'll learn about the underlying causes of insomnia as well as other sleep disorders and about the environmental, lifestyle, physiological, and psychological factors that play roles in sleep enhancement and disruption. You'll also discover a variety of nutritional and herbal supplements that provide safe, effective alternatives to the drugs that are frequently prescribed as sleep-aids. Learning about your sleep problem is an important first step toward resolving it; the information you find here should be everything you need to help you get a good night's rest.

Why a Good Night's Sleep Is Essential for Your Health

S leep is a curious physiological phenomenon. Although there's no question that sleep is essential—as necessary to our health and survival as food, water, and air—scientists still don't know exactly why we sleep, even after decades of high-tech research. It's no secret, however, that sufficient sleep is necessary to feel physically energetic and mentally alert. In addition, sleep appears to help restore proper levels of neurotransmitters in the brain and to play a role in emotional well-being. Some scientists theorize that the process of dreaming helps us to organize and preserve memories.

Despite sleep's enduring mysteries, one thing is clear: we need a good night's sleep to feel and be at our best. In this chapter, you'll learn about normal sleep patterns and requirements, problems of sleep disruption, and the costs of sleep deprivation.

THE GROSS ANATOMY OF SLEEP

Carefully conducted studies have shown that most adults seem to need about eight hours of sleep in each twenty-four-hour period. Most people are naturally active during the day and sleep at night and it's also normal to experience a period of sleepiness at midday, which in many cultures is sanctioned with a siesta. The cycle of sleeping and waking is determined by an internal biological clock that sets circadian rhythms ("circadian" means "about a day"). In addition to regulating the sleep/wake cycle, this internal clock controls the timing of hundreds of metabolic and other bodily functions.

The light that enters the eyes plays a key role in setting circadian rhythms. Light travels from the retinas as electrical signals through the optic nerves toward the center of the brain and reaches the hypothalamus, the body's master clock, which contains a tiny cluster of nerves called the suprachiasmatic nucleus (SCN). As daylight wanes each day, the SCN signals another structure in the brain, the pineal gland, to produce melatonin, a hormone that promotes the onset of sleep. Conversely, at sunrise, the pineal gland is signaled by the SCN to decrease its production of melatonin, thereby promoting wakefulness. The hypothalamus coordinates the sleep/wake cycle with a host of other circadian rhythms, like the rise and fall of body temperature and the release of various other hormones, throughout every twenty-four-hour period.

Various other internal and external factors can impinge on these rhythms and the resulting circadian disturbance may be most noticeable for its impact on sleep. For example, hormonal shifts (such as those of menopause) can wreak havoc with the sleep/wake cycle; traveling across time zones is well known for turning normal sleep patterns upside down; and even light exposure at the wrong time—whether from a full moon or an artificial source—can disrupt sleep by incorrectly resetting the internal clock.

The Stages of Sleep

It's helpful to understand the progression of normal sleep in order to gain a better understanding of why sleep disorders are so disruptive to health and well-being. Since the 1950s, scientists have used polysomnography, which is the simultaneous recording of electrophysiological and other data during sleep, to probe the activities of the sleeping brain and body. Five distinct stages occur during sleep and each plays an essential role in helping you to feel well rested and alert when you awaken. Four of these stages are classified as non-REM (or NREM) and the fifth as REM sleep. REM, as you may already know, stands for rapid eye movement.

Light Non-REM Sleep

Stage one, also called the hypnagogic state, is a light non-REM stage that is the transition between wakefulness and sleep. During stage one, external stimuli fade into the background and your thoughts become unfocused as you drift in and out of consciousness. Your muscles relax and your body temperature, blood pressure, and heart rate slowly begin to decrease.

Brain waves in stage one are rapid and irregular. The majority are theta waves, at a frequency of 4–7 cycles per second. Intermittent alpha waves, which have a frequency of 8–13 cycles per second and indicate relaxed wakefulness, can also be seen on the polysomnographic recording. Levels of serotonin, a neurotransmitter that enables communication between nerve cells and acts as a natural tranquilizer, begin to increase in the brain during this stage.

For most people with healthy sleep patterns, stage one sleep lasts only for a few minutes. When stage two of non-REM sleep takes over, relaxation deepens. Brain waves in stage two become larger and show erratic bursts of electrical activity such as sleep spindles and K-complexes, which are waveforms named for their characteristic appearance on the polysomnograph. Although not much happens in the way of physical restoration during stage one sleep, some physical repair processes begin during stage two.

Deep Non-REM Sleep

It's more difficult to awaken a sleeper during the deep sleep that follows stages one and two. As you move into non-REM stages three and four, brain waves become very large and slow and are called delta waves, with a low frequency of $1/_2$–4 cycles per second. In general, between 20 and 50 percent of the brain activity recorded in stage three consists of delta waves; during stage four, more than 50 percent is delta waves, with the remainder theta waves.

Although a sleeper in one or the other of these stages appears simply to be breathing slowly and regularly and lying mostly still, deep non-REM sleep is essential for health. This quiet, restorative time provides the opportunity for the brain and nervous system to bring the body's systems back into balance and for the body to do most of its repair work.

Good-quality sleep is largely defined by the percentage of time spent in stage four, which is also called delta sleep. Researchers have yet to determine the optimal amount of delta sleep but there's no question that this sleep stage contributes significantly to our health and well-being. During delta sleep, immune function is strengthened, red blood cells are renewed, and growth hormone is secreted; growth hormone is not only critical for the healthy development of children but also for the repair of muscle tissue in adults. People who are chronically deprived of delta sleep often suffer from an increased incidence of illness as well as general aches, pains, and fatigue.

REM Sleep

After about an hour of the non-REM stages, sleep shifts into an active stage characterized by rapid eye movements (REMs). In REM sleep, your brain waves appear very similar to those of wakefulness but you're actually dreaming. The nerves that control body movement are also temporarily suppressed by the brain's inhibition of certain neurons in the spinal cord, which prevents you (for the most part) from physically acting out your dreams. During this stage, heart rate, blood pressure, respiration, and gastric secretions increase.

Although infants spend approximately 50 percent of their total sleep time in the REM stage, the amount of REM sleep generally decreases with age. As an adult, you spend about three-quarters of your sleeping time in non-REM sleep and only during the remaining quarter are you actively dreaming. REM sleep occurs several times throughout a normal night, as we enter into a REM period about every ninety minutes while sleeping. A typical REM period lasts approximately twenty to forty minutes but can increase in length to as much as an hour if the sleep session has been several hours or longer.

The exact function of REM sleep is not understood but there seems to be a definite need for it. Studies have demonstrated that it's during the REM stage that memories are organized and stored, which is an essential component of learning. The dreams that characterize REM sleep also appear to provide an avenue for working out problems on conscious and subconscious levels. Although most dreams are forgotten soon after awakening, deprivation of REM sleep and dreams can lead to irritability, anxiety, confusion, and problems with impulse control.

HOW MUCH SLEEP DO YOU NEED?

In a 2001 poll, the National Sleep Foundation found that 63 percent of American adults were getting less than eight hours of sleep per night; most people were averaging about seven hours a night but 31 percent of adults regularly fell short of even this amount. By comparison, people living in the early 1900s regularly slept nine hours or more per night. The advent of electricity has played a major role in shifting sleep patterns. Prior to electric lighting, people tended to go to bed when it got dark. The availability of bright light at the flick of a switch has undoubtedly shortened the sleep period and also shifted its timing. Without darkness, the brain's production of melatonin is inhibited, which results in a tendency to stay up far past dusk.

Most of us have been told throughout our adult lives that we need eight hours of sleep per night—but the reality is that some people seem to thrive on only six hours of sleep, whereas others need nine hours or more in order to function optimally. Clearly, there are individual differences when it comes to defining "enough" sleep. Perhaps the best indicator of whether or not you are getting enough sleep is how you feel when you're awake. If you wake up in the morning without an alarm clock and feel refreshed and reasonably energetic, then you're likely getting enough sleep.

Variations in Sleep Patterns

Researchers have found that people who thrive on less sleep, referred to as "short sleepers," spend a proportionally larger amount of their sleep time in REM and stage four, which are considered to be the most restorative stages. "Long sleepers," on the other hand, who generally require nine or more hours of sleep, spend a proportionally greater amount of their sleep time in stage two, which is a much lighter stage. Women also tend to sleep more than men do, although the reason for this gender difference is unclear.

For most of us, the biological clock operates on a cycle of roughly twenty-four hours. However, not only do people differ in the amount of sleep they require, they also differ in when they naturally want to sleep within that cycle. Some people are most energetic early in the day; these "larks" consistently rise early in the morning, no matter what time they may have gone to bed. Others are naturally "night owls" who don't feel at their best until late evening. But even with these variations in specific sleep patterns, most people do become sleepy at some point after dark, particularly between midnight and dawn.

Although sleep patterns seem to have a genetic basis, many additional factors influence sleep needs. If you're sick, for example, you need more rest to help your immune system function properly in its fight against illness. Regular physical exercise can reduce the amount of sleep you normally require but rigorous or unaccustomed exercise can increase your sleep need and exercising too close to bedtime can interfere with your sleep (see Chapter 10).

The amount of sleep an individual needs usually changes over the lifespan. Infants and children sleep longer and more deeply than adults; in fact, infants can sleep as much as eighteen hours per day. With age, sleep tends to become lighter and more easily disrupted and people often find that they sleep less than when they were younger. However, these changes often result from the emergence of sleep disorders (particularly in the elderly), not from a decreased need for sleep. On the other hand, if you find that you consistently need more sleep than you did earlier in life, it's probably because the caliber of your sleep is not as good as it once was. Sleep quality is just as important as the actual number of hours spent sleeping.

Despite individual sleep pattern variations, getting enough sleep—and getting good-quality sleep—is essential for everyone's optimal physical and emotional well-being. The trend in our society, unfortunately, has been to devalue sleep, packing as many activities as possible into each day and leaving little time for rest. Over the past century, the average amount of sleep time in the United States has been reduced by 20 percent and the result of this deficit is that we are a nation of sleep-deprived people. Even though our way of life has changed, our bodies still need adequate sleep.

SLEEP IS NOT OPTIONAL

Many people believe that if they routinely sleep less, their bodies and brains will then become accustomed to sleep restriction and be able to function as before on fewer hours of sleep; researchers have found, however, that this wishful notion isn't true. In fact, a recent study reported in the journal *Sleep* demonstrated that getting fewer than six hours of sleep for several nights in a row impaired mental and physical performance as much as not sleeping at all for two consecutive nights.

Hans P.A. Van Dongen, an assistant professor at the University of Pennsylvania School of Medicine in Philadelphia, studied forty-eight people who were divided into four groups: one each that slept four, six, or eight hours a night for two weeks and one that went without sleep for three days and two nights. (All participants were monitored to ensure that they didn't nap or use caffeine during the study.) In addition to undergoing a variety of mental and physiological tests each day, the participants self-evaluated their level of fatigue. The research team found that the three groups of people who slept less than eight hours per night had slower reaction times and were less able to think clearly and perform simple memory tasks. Although the participants whose sleep was restricted for two weeks reported feeling less tired than those who went without sleep altogether for two nights, the results showed that they performed just as poorly on the tests.

Hazards of Too Little Sleep

Psychosomatic complaints such as headaches, gastrointestinal upset, and loss of appetite are frequent side effects of insufficient sleep. Sleep deprivation also has a significant effect on psychological states, both cognitive and emotional. One of the first indications of insufficient sleep is difficulty with concentration and short-term memory. Thinking processes slow down, reaction time gets longer, and creativity wanes. Even being short-changed an hour or two of sleep at night decreases problem-solving capacity the next day, because decision-making and judgment depend on alertness.

Most sleep-deprived people also tend to become irritable, which causes tension with family members, friends, and co-workers and greatly increases the potential for conflict. More disturbing psychological manifestations of sleep deprivation resemble serious mental illnesses such as psychosis, paranoia, and schizophrenia. Researchers have observed that it's not at all uncommon for a sleep-deprived person to exhibit sporadic episodes of bizarre behaviors: for example, paranoia, delusions of grandeur, hallucinations, and personality changes including aggression.

Because sleep is a necessity and not an option, "microsleeps" can occur if you aren't getting sufficient rest. A microsleep is a brief period of time—generally just a few seconds—when the brain enters a sleep state, usually without the person's awareness; during these involuntary lapses in attention, the person loses conscious control of thoughts and actions and has no recall of anything that takes place during the episode. Not surprisingly, the incidence of microsleeps increases in direct proportion to lack of sleep. Microsleeps occur regardless of whatever activity you may be involved in and these black-outs can be extremely dangerous: for example, if they happen while you're driving or operating machinery.

Clearly, a lack of sleep puts us and those around us at risk, sometimes with catastrophic consequences. Well-known sleep-related industrial accidents in recent history include the incident at Three Mile Island's nuclear plant in 1979, the disastrous nuclear explosion at Chernobyl in 1986, and the *Exxon Valdez* oil spill off the coast of Alaska in 1989. In the United States, it's estimated that sleep-related accidents cost about $56 billion annually. More tragically, 25,000 lives are lost each year in accidents related to sleep deprivation. According to the National Highway Traffic Safety Administration, more than 100,000 traffic accidents every year are caused by overtired drivers.

Even if sleep deprivation doesn't result in an accident, it has many other negative outcomes. Sleep is the primary time when the body performs many restorative functions including detoxification, repairing cellular damage, and searching out and destroying foreign invaders. A lack of sleep wears down the body, decreasing levels of important immune system compounds, which results in lowered immunity and more frequent infections.

Even premature aging is linked to insufficient sleep. In a study at the University of Chicago, researchers found significant physiological deterioration in healthy participants (aged eighteen to twenty-seven) after only six days of cutting back from eight hours of sleep per night to four hours; the participants were found to take 40 percent longer than normal to regulate their blood sugar and their ability to produce and regulate insulin dropped to 30 percent below normal. The researchers concluded that getting too little sleep negatively affects the body's regulation of blood glucose and insulin levels. Poor control of blood sugar and insulin is now recognized as a primary factor in chronic degenerative diseases such as diabetes, hypertension, cardiovascular disease, obesity, and memory impairment.

How Sleep Debt Affects You

Sleep debt is the difference between the hours of sleep that you need and the hours of sleep that you're actually getting. You begin to accumulate a sleep debt with any more than a night or two of insufficient sleep, even if you seem able to function on just a few hours of sleep per night. The costs of a sleep debt, as mentioned previously, are high, especially for the brain; brain activity becomes less efficient, resulting in memory problems and difficulty performing routine tasks.

In fact, your body may be able to get by on less sleep than your brain, because both the length and composition of sleep are factors in whether your brain incurs a sleep debt. The brain is active and performs important functions during sleep, particularly during REM periods, when it processes information taken in during the day and moves the data from short-term memory to long-term memory. REM sleep is also the brain's most restorative sleep stage, when supplies of various neurotransmitters are replenished (in contrast to non-REM sleep, when the emphasis of restore and repair is on the rest of the body). REM periods lengthen over the course of a night's sleep, with the longest REM period between the seventh and eighth hours; therefore, if you sleep less than eight hours, your brain is missing out on its most refreshing and rejuvenating hour of sleep.

Unfortunately, you can't repay a sleep debt by simply "sleeping in" on the weekend. If you lose an hour or two of sleep one night, you can probably make up for it with a couple extra hours of sleep the following night. If you routinely undersleep, then you need several weeks of consistently sleeping eight or more hours per night to begin restoring your body and brain to healthy, normal functioning. The truth is that you can never completely make up for all of your lost sleep—but acknowledging that you probably need more sleep than you're getting is a good place to begin resolving your sleep debt. For the millions of people struggling with insomnia and other sleep problems, however, chronic sleep deprivation and mounting sleep debt are a painful reality.

2

Insomnia and Its Primary Causes

Almost everyone has had occasional trouble sleeping. A stressful day, too much caffeine, a barking dog, or the excitement of leaving on a trip can all interfere with a good night's sleep. Consider the following inset, which lists symptoms of the sleep disorder known as insomnia. Do any—or several—of these statements apply to you or to a loved one?

In combating insomnia and its effects, approximately 70 million Americans spend close to $150 million annually on remedies to help them sleep—or to keep them awake during the day after a bout of sleeplessness. This chapter describes some of the most common causes of insomnia and also provides insight into how you can treat these problems naturally.

Symptoms of Insomnia

- I have trouble falling asleep when I go to bed at night.
- It takes me at least twenty minutes to fall asleep when I go to bed.
- I awaken during the night and can't get back to sleep.
- I awaken earlier in the morning than I would like.
- I worry about being able to get a good night's sleep.
- I don't feel refreshed when I awaken in the morning.
- I feel sleepy during the day.
- I use stimulants like caffeine to keep myself alert during the day.

WHAT IS INSOMNIA?

Insomnia comes in a variety of frequencies and forms. Some people have difficulty falling asleep, while others can go to sleep without a problem at first but then awaken persistently during the night. If you sometimes have trouble sleeping, you can count yourself among the one-third of Americans who experience a disturbed or even sleepless night once in a while. But for millions of people in the United States (and elsewhere), a peaceful night's sleep is a rare occurrence; it's estimated that at least 10 percent of Americans suffer from recurring insomnia.

Insomnia can be either acute or chronic. Acute insomnia occurs only occasionally. It is transient, generally lasting for only a few nights or up to a month at the most. Acute insomnia is most often due to some type of emotional stress or excitement. For example, financial worries or a fight with your spouse can keep you awake at night—as can receiving a promotion or anticipating a vacation. Temporary physical discomfort such as that from the flu or a sore back can also lead to short-term insomnia. Jet lag can produce acute insomnia because the body's internal clock can't always adjust right away to a different time zone. Even exercise, which is undeniably a healthy habit, can cause this type of sleep problem if the activity is too vigorous within about three hours of bedtime. In cases of acute insomnia, the body quickly returns to a normal sleeping pattern when the underlying emotional or physical issue is resolved.

Chronic insomnia, however, is quite different; it persists for more than a month and can even continue for years. It's rare for someone to have trouble sleeping every night but it's not unusual for people with chronic insomnia to suffer from disrupted sleep at least three nights a week. The National Sleep Foundation estimates that, on average, people with chronic insomnia have problems sleeping about sixteen nights out of every thirty. Chronic insomnia has many causes, from underlying physical problems such as arthritis or breathing disorders to long-term emotional stress. Even simple environmental or lifestyle factors (see the next section) can contribute to chronic sleep difficulties.

Insomnia—both acute and chronic—tends to affect older people more often than younger people and women seem to be more prone to having problems sleeping than men. Many people assume that sleep disorders are primarily caused by anxiety or depression. It's true that people who are stressed, anxious, or depressed often have problems sleeping (see Psy-

Typical Causes of Acute Insomnia

- Short-term emotional stress
- Excessive use of caffeine, alcohol, or tobacco
- Environmental disturbances (such as noise, light, or temperature extremes)
- Disturbance of normal sleep/wake cycle (such as jet lag)
- Side effects from medications (including some painkillers, cold and allergy remedies, and antidepressants)

Typical Causes of Chronic Insomnia

- Medical conditions (such as gastroesophageal reflux)
- Prolonged emotional stress or emotional disorders (such as depression or anxiety)
- Sleep disorders (such as sleep apnea or restless legs syndrome)
- Chronic use of caffeine, alcohol, or tobacco
- Poor sleep habits
- Disturbance of normal sleep/wake cycle (such as shift work)
- Certain (long-term) medications (including decongestants and some antidepressants)

chophysiological Factors in Insomnia on page 19), but the majority of people who suffer from insomnia do not have an actual mood disorder. Ongoing insomnia, however, can definitely cause extreme fatigue, anxiety over not being able to sleep, and eventually depression. During stressful times, you may be able to help yourself get a good night's sleep by using the relaxation techniques, nutritional supplements, and herbs discussed in this book.

ENVIRONMENTAL AND LIFESTYLE FACTORS IN INSOMNIA

Some of us are more susceptible than others to sleep difficulties. We're all hardwired differently and certain individuals are more sensitive to disturbances in their external—or internal—environment. For example, while light sleepers may be awakened by the slightest noise, other people are able to sleep through virtually anything. Many lifestyle and environmental factors, from a loud neighbor to a lack of exercise, can interfere with a good night's sleep. Addressing these issues is sometimes all that's needed to restore a healthful sleeping pattern.

Diet and Exercise Affect Sleep

What we eat and drink can significantly influence our sleep for better or for worse, yet this seemingly obvious point is frequently overlooked. Caffeine is at the top of the list of dietary sleep disrupters—even the residual amounts of caffeine in decaffeinated coffee and tea can cause sleep problems for some people. This stimulant is widely used to temporarily delay the onset of sleep and even if it doesn't do that, it often leads to awakening during the night (see Caffeine and Insomnia on page 56). Caffeine is especially likely to cause insomnia when ingested in the late afternoon or evening but caffeine used at any time of day can contribute to sleep disturbance in people who are sensitive to its effects.

Alcohol, usually considered to be more of a sedative than a stimulant, can cause sleep problems as well. Its initial effects are relaxing but it has stimulating effects once it's metabolized by the body. Although a glass of wine with dinner may promote relaxation, too much alcohol (more than a drink or two per day) can contribute to both acute and chronic insomnia. Drinking alcohol within a couple of hours of bedtime is especially likely to cause sleep disturbances (see Subtle Sleep Disrupters on page 55).

Nicotine, an even more powerful stimulant than caffeine, is another common contributor to insomnia. Studies have shown nicotine to cause difficulties in falling asleep, restlessness during the night, nightmares, problems awakening in the morning, and daytime sleepiness. Smokers also suffer from a greater incidence of sleep-related breathing disorders such as snoring (see also Sleep Apnea on page 26) than do nonsmokers. It's helpful to realize that people who use tobacco over the course of the day—and people who try to quit—experience nicotine withdrawal after they've gone to bed, which can cause awakenings during the night as well as tension and anxiety that contribute to sleeplessness; fortunately, these withdrawal symptoms tend to subside after about ten days of abstaining from nicotine. Stopping tobacco use improves sleep quality and overall well-being.

The amount of food that you eat, as well as when you eat it, are often directly related to restless or disturbed sleep. Having a large meal too close to bedtime, for example, can make it difficult to fall asleep at first. On the other hand, eating too little during the day can lead to insomnia later, because a nighttime drop in blood sugar level can trigger awakening. Many dietary factors, in fact, play a role in ensuring a good night's sleep. (See Chapter 4 for more information about creating a diet that includes helpful nutrients and eliminates food stressors.)

One reason that people tend to suffer more from sleep problems as they get older may be that insufficient physical activity can contribute to insomnia. Regular daily exercise (such as a thirty-minute brisk walk in the morning or afternoon) is an excellent health habit that also promotes restful sleep at night. As with food intake, however, remember that type, amount, and timing may determine whether your exercise is beneficial or detrimental to your sleep. Vigorous exercise within three to four hours of bedtime can be overly stimulating and trigger wakefulness, whereas slower, meditative movements such as gentle stretching and breathing exercises can help calm the body and mind and make it easier to go to sleep (see Chapter 10).

Your Surroundings and Your Sleep

For most people, quiet, dark, and peaceful surroundings are necessary for restful sleep—but whether your bedroom is in the city or the country, environmental disruptions often intrude on slumber. Traffic sounds, barking dogs, television in another room, trains, airplanes, or a snoring bed partner can all disturb your sleep, even if they don't awaken you. If there is noise in your environment that you can't control, consider investing in a sound machine, which masks external noise with a peaceful sound such as a gentle rain or ocean waves. Even the sound of an electric fan can be soothing and is excellent for blocking out bothersome noise.

Light is another primary environmental contributor to insomnia. The distraction of streetlights, lamplight from a neighboring house, or even the moon shining through your bedroom window can make it difficult to sleep. Also, as discussed in Chapter 1, darkness is a physiological trigger for sleep onset and even a small amount of light can reset circadian rhythms and signal the body to wake up. Make your bedroom as dark as possible with blinds, shades, or drapes that block out all light at night. An eye mask (available at pharmacies) provides a simple and portable solution to a sleep problem caused by light interference.

Consider whether your bedroom may be too hot or too cold, as a comfortable temperature is essential for a good night's sleep. A slightly cool room generally promotes the most restful sleep; most people sleep best within a temperature range of 60–65°F (16–18°C). During the winter, lower the heat in your house at night and layer your bed with sheets, blankets, and comforters so you can easily make yourself warmer or cooler as desired. If possible, sleep with your windows open to allow fresh air to circulate. During the summer, air conditioning at night may be essential for sleeping well in a hot or humid climate.

People differ in the sort of bed that they find most comfortable and a mattress that is too soft or too hard is a common contributor to sleep problems. The best way to discover your ideal sleep surface is to visit a retailer and try out various mattresses until you find the right combination of support and comfort. A good-quality mattress and foundation (box spring) supports the shoulders, hips, and lower back, which are the heaviest parts of the body. Inadequate support can cause chronic back pain but a very firm mattress isn't necessarily the answer, because a surface that is too rigid can create uncomfortable pressure points and soreness. Many mattresses provide firm support and also have a layer of cushioning on top for optimal comfort. In choosing a sleep set, don't overlook size as a factor in comfort. If you sleep with a partner, choose a queen- or king-size bed for adequate freedom of movement during the night. You should probably replace your mattress and foundation at least every ten years to ensure comfortable rest.

Sleep Problems of Modern Life

An erratic schedule, so common nowadays, is also a common cause of sleep problems that can progress to become full-fledged sleep disorders. Most people are aware that changing time zones or working the night shift interferes with the body's natural sleep/wake cycle. Many don't realize, however, that the common pattern of staying up late on weekend nights and "sleeping in" on weekend mornings can be just as disruptive to sleep and circadian rhythms. In general, the body thrives on a regular schedule; establishing a regular time for sleeping and waking is helpful for both preventing and overcoming sleep disorders.

Jet Lag

If you've ever traveled to another time zone, you've most likely experienced sleep disturbance as a consequence. When your internal clock must suddenly reset itself to a different schedule, the disorientation, irritability, fatigue, and insomnia characteristic of jet lag may result. Flying across time zones requires adjusting the mechanisms that regulate body temperature, heart rate, hormone levels, and sleep pattern and it usually takes at least a couple of days for your body to normalize. The more time zones crossed, the more severe jet lag tends to be.

If at all possible, schedule your flight during the day. This enables you, after arriving at your destination, to have dinner and go to bed on the local schedule, which will help you adjust more quickly. Avoid the impulse to nap, as daytime napping will only make it more difficult for you to sleep during the local nighttime. Instead, one of the most beneficial things you can do is to exercise as soon as possible after your arrival. It's a good idea, in fact, to take a brisk thirty-minute walk every day while traveling (see Chapter 10). If you walk in the morning, you'll adjust even more quickly to local time, because the sunlight exposure will help reset your biological clock.

Several other natural approaches can be taken to counteract the effects of jet lag. Siberian ginseng will help your body adjust more quickly to the stresses of travel (see Chapter 4). To help settle down before bed, take the herbal relaxant passionflower, which calms the nervous system and promotes sleep (see Chapter 5), or the hormone melatonin, which signals your body that it's time to go to sleep (see Chapter 8). Using essential oils for nighttime relaxation and for enhanced energy and mental clarity during the daytime (see Chapter 11) can also ease the strain of traveling and help you adjust to a new time zone with a minimum of stress.

Shift Work

Shift workers are especially susceptible to chronic insomnia because they often switch work schedules every week or two and tend to follow yet another schedule on their days off. To add to the problem, people typically have increasing difficulty adjusting to these scheduling irregularities as they get older.

The disruptive effects of shift work on sleep can be somewhat minimized by systematically rotating shifts forward (that is, going from morning, to evening, to night) instead of working according to a randomly changing schedule of shifts. It's helpful to maintain the same shift for at least three weeks, which gives the body time to adjust to the variation. Although it may be difficult, it is beneficial for shift workers to try to maintain their current work schedule during their time off as well, even on weekends and holidays. It is also very important for the shift worker to allot a sufficient period of time for sleep—maybe eight hours, maybe a bit more or a bit less, depending on individual need—so that body and brain can cycle through all of the various sleep stages and perform the necessary tasks of repair and restoration.

If shift work is contributing to your insomnia, make sure that when you go to bed your bedroom is completely dark and quiet, to cue your body that it's time to rest and to trigger the secretion of the "sleep hormone" melatonin. Practicing relaxation techniques (such as those described in Chapters 10 and 11) can help your body and mind calm down after work to allow for restful sleep. Taking supplemental melatonin (see Chapter 8) or herbal sedatives such as passionflower and valerian (see Chapter 6) can also help promote sleep onset. In addition, maintaining a healthful diet and exercising regularly will help mitigate some of the stressful effects of shift work. Avoid excessive amounts of caffeine; if you must use it, be sure to completely avoid it within several hours of going to bed (see Chapter 4).

PSYCHOPHYSIOLOGICAL FACTORS IN INSOMNIA

Of all the contributors to insomnia, stress is the most common underlying theme. Stress is simply the body's heightened physiological response to the ever-changing conditions of life. Relationship difficulties, job pressures, family problems, and financial concerns are some typical sources of stress but the stress response can also be triggered by more joyful experiences such as a new love relationship, a move, or a work promotion. We generally interpret positive stressors as pleasant, exciting experiences but they can create anxiety just as negative stressors can.

An event or situation doesn't inherently cause stress: the interpretation of it and response to it do. People vary in their ability to cope with change or adverse circumstances and what one person finds devastating might not upset another at all. There are, of course, difficult and tragic life events that cause most people to feel distress. But for the most part, the situations that generate stress in our lives are minor annoyances that we allow to consume us. The physiological changes triggered by stress occur largely beneath our conscious awareness, so we may not even be aware of what is happening within ourselves until the tension erupts into a headache, backache, upset stomach, racing heart, or sleepless night.

The Impact of Stress

When we are anxious, we react physically as though danger is imminent. The autonomic nervous system (the neurons that control involuntary functions such as heart rate, blood pressure, respiration, and digestion) is aroused, which speeds up heart rate and breathing, raises blood pressure, dumps stored sugars (in the form of glucose) into the bloodstream, and increases the adrenal glands' production of stress hormones such as adrenaline and cortisol. Dubbed the "fight-or-flight response," this reaction is an automatic, life-saving instinct that evolved at the dawn of human history when, in order to survive, we needed the ability to either fight for our lives or run away from danger. The physiological changes that occur during this stress response supply the burst of energy and strength to deal with life-threatening danger. But our bodies don't usually distinguish between life-threatening danger and ordinary stressors such as job pressures and financial worries.

Whether unconscious or not, stress—especially chronic, unresolved stress—takes a significant toll on your physical and emotional well-being. Insomnia is only one of the numerous symptoms and conditions related to stress. In fact, as many as 90 percent of all illnesses are deemed to be stress related. If you suffer from fatigue, anxiety, diarrhea, headache, back pain, rapid heart rate, irritability, muscle tension, stomach upset, teeth grinding, loss of sexual interest, difficulty concentrating, or insomnia, you should consider stress as a suspect.

Adding fuel to the fire, the ways we deal with stress are often unhealthful. Using alcohol or other drugs, smoking, overeating, and watching too much television are just a few of the negative coping mechanisms that are so prevalent in our society. It's likely that you've learned some negative coping patterns for handling stress but there are many positive ways that you can learn to manage life stressors. Creating a healthful lifestyle builds a strong foundation that enables you to meet the challenges of life with a minimum of wear and tear on your body and psyche. A nutrient-rich diet (see Chapter 4), regular exercise (see Chapter 10), and plenty of rest enhance your physical resistance to illness and fatigue. Learning new coping skills such as overcoming negative thinking patterns (see Chapter 9) or practicing calming techniques such as deep relaxation and meditation (see Chapters 10 and 11) help bolster your emotional well-being.

Herbs can also be powerful allies against the stresses in our lives. Vitality-building herbs such as Siberian ginseng (see Herbs for Better Sleep on page 51) support the endocrine system, the body's network of hormone-producing glands. The endocrine system works with the nervous system to control various physiological functions including response to stressors. Mildly relaxing herbs such as chamomile and lemon balm can be used to promote a sense of calm (see Chapter 5). Stronger sedative and mood-elevating herbs such as kava can be taken on a short-term basis to relax the mind and body (see Chapter 6) so that the deeper cognitive and behavioral work of understanding emotional turmoil or learning new ways of coping can take place (see Chapter 9).

Stress and Insomnia

We're all subject to a variety of potential stressors in any given day. Problems at work, financial worries, and relationship challenges can make it difficult to get a peaceful night's rest. But because not all of us react to stress in the same way, a life event that causes insomnia for one person may not affect the sleep of another individual at all. Two things, however, are certain across the board: first, that stress hormones produced by the adrenal glands result in a state of vigilant alertness; and secondly, that if you're feeling stressed enough that your glands increase their output of these hormones, you're not likely to sleep peacefully. Scientists have attempted to unravel the role that stress plays in sleeping patterns and also to discover who is susceptible to stress-induced insomnia and why.

In a study of the relationship of stress to insomnia, researchers at Pennsylvania State University enlisted eleven insomniacs and thirteen healthy sleepers to spend four nights in the College of Medicine's Sleep Research and Treatment Center. During the fourth day and night, each participant's blood was sampled every half-hour in order to measure levels of cortisol and adrenocorticotropin (a pituitary hormone that promotes the release of more cortisol). Both the daytime and nighttime blood samples from the group of insomniacs contained significantly higher levels of these two stress hormones than the samples from the group of healthy sleepers. According to the researchers, the findings in the insomniacs point to chronic hyperarousal of the central nervous system, which not only causes insomnia but also increases the risk of anxiety, depression, and physiological disorders (such as hypertension) associated with chronic stress. They concluded that managing stress levels is necessary to improve sleep, overall health, and well-being.

Another study, this time in Quebec at Université Laval, Sainte-Foy, investigated the interrelationship of stress, coping skills, and sleep patterns. The researchers enlisted sixty-seven individuals: forty suffering from insomnia and twenty-seven healthy sleepers. Over a period of twenty-one days, the participants were asked to keep track of daily stressful life events, degree of presleep arousal, and quality and amount of sleep; they were also evaluated by the researchers for depression, anxiety, stressful life events, and coping skills. Interestingly, though the two groups reported similar numbers of stressful life events, their perception of these stressors differed significantly. The insomniacs consistently perceived their lives as more stressful than did the healthy sleepers, which was reflected by nighttime sleep patterns showing poorer sleep quality for those who reported more stress. The researchers concluded that the perception of a lack of control over stressful events predisposes an individual to insomnia more than the actual events do and suggested that treatment for insomnia should include education in coping with life stressors.

Clearly, the ability to cope with stressors can make all the difference between insomnia and a peaceful night's sleep. Unfortunately, insomnia can be a stressor in itself. If you sleep poorly for a few nights, you may begin to worry about not being able to sleep, which sets the stage for insomnia to become a learned pattern. Trying too hard to go to sleep triggers more worry and stress and the process of going to bed can become an anxiety-provoking experience; even the rituals associated with bedtime— putting on your pajamas, turning off the lights, and getting into bed—can trigger feelings of anxiety. (This phenomenon explains why some people who find it impossible to get a good night's sleep in their own bed can fall asleep easily on the sofa or when traveling and sleeping in a different bed.)

This type of insomnia, called learned insomnia, can be remedied by improving sleep habits and learning specific techniques to reduce anxiety (see Chapter 9). Herbal and nutritional supplements can also be used to relieve anxiety and promote the internal calmness that allows sleep to occur (see Chapters 4–8). For all stress-related cases of insomnia, practicing relaxation techniques such as those described in this book (see Chapters 10 and 11) will help clear the mind and set the stage for a good night's sleep.

Beyond Stress: Anxiety and Depression

Everyone has experienced temporary anxiety in reaction to a stressful situation. When a transient anxiety-provoking situation passes, so does the fight-or-flight response that it evokes. The autonomic nervous system calms down and all body systems return to a relaxed state of functioning. This resting stage is crucial for physical and emotional health. For many people, however, anxiety takes on a life of its own and becomes an underlying current of unrest that interferes with normal living. Although the body can handle short-term and clearly defined stressors pretty easily, problems arise with long-term stressors such as relationship, job, family, or money problems that create a chronic state of anxiety. Anxiety that is chronic or severe causes wear-and-tear on the body and the psyche and has a significant detrimental effect on health.

Common symptoms of anxiety include insomnia, heart palpitations, feelings of tightness in the chest, breathing difficulties, chest pain, headaches, muscle spasms, back pain, dizziness, digestive disturbances, fear, and the nagging feeling that something bad is going to happen. Anxiety can range in severity from mild nervousness to severe panic attacks and phobias; whatever your level of anxiety, it is always a signal that you are in distress and that you need to pay attention to your physical and emotional well-being.

Many doctors prescribe tranquilizers for anxiety and its accompanying insomnia. While these drugs are effective, they are also extremely addictive and usually require increasingly larger doses over time to have a relaxing effect. Pharmaceutical tranquilizers also have serious side effects such as mental confusion and grogginess and can cause rebound anxiety (that is, an increase in anxiety when the treatment is discontinued). Non-drug approaches like relaxation training, meditation, and yoga are often effective for mild to moderate anxiety. They have no negative side effects and give you skills for coping with stress. Because anxiety is often caused by a feeling of loss of control, learning to manage stress in this way is empowering.

If you have a more intense manifestation of anxiety such as a phobia (when a specific object or activity elicits extreme fear) or panic attacks (severe, spontaneous attacks of anxiety that occur unpredictably along with feelings of doom and fears of dying or going crazy), seek professional help. Some health problems such as hypoglycemia, thyroid disorders, and hormonal imbalances associated with premenstrual syndrome and menopause can trigger anxiety. If your anxiety is severe or chronic or if you do not feel better after following the suggestions in this book, consult your healthcare practitioner.

Depression is frequently associated with persistent problems in falling asleep, difficulty in staying asleep, or early morning awakening. Sleep disturbance, though, is not the only sign of depression, which is usually accompanied by other symptoms such as a loss of interest in activities that were previously enjoyed, change in appetite (eating more or less than usual), and irritability or sadness. If you suffer from symptoms of a mood disorder for more than a couple of weeks, it's important to consult your doctor or a psychotherapist. Treating the underlying depression or anxiety is essential for alleviating the insomnia associated with a mood disorder.

Ironically, many of the medications used for treating depression and anxiety can disrupt sleep patterns. Most of the newer antidepressants such as Prozac, Zoloft, Paxil, and other selective serotonin-reuptake inhibitors (SSRIs) can have significant stimulating effects for some people. Although these drugs are often prescribed for insomnia (see Chapter 12), they may actually cause sleep disturbances themselves. St. John's wort, an herbal alternative to pharmaceutical antidepressants, does not cause overstimulation and, in fact, can be helpful for treating insomnia that is related to depression or anxiety (see Chapter 7).

3

Other Sleep Disorders and Sleep Problems

Avariety of physical and psychological conditions—some unusual, some so ordinary that we take them for granted—can contribute to sleep problems. In men, for example, prostate enlargement can disrupt sleep by necessitating frequent urination during the night. For women, the hormonal shifts and accompanying hot flashes of menopause are a common cause of insomnia. Among the numerous medical problems that cause significant sleep disruption are sleep apnea, restless legs syndrome, gastroesophageal reflux, chronic pain, and psychiatric disorders such as anxiety and depression.

Insomnia caused by another underlying disorder is referred to as secondary insomnia. A few nights of sleeplessness generally isn't cause for concern but if you've been having trouble sleeping for several weeks, a visit to a doctor is a good idea. It's important to check with your physician to identify or rule out any other health problems that may be at the root of your sleep difficulty. In a case of serious medical or psychiatric illness, treating the primary disorder is essential to resolving the secondary insomnia.

You'll learn in this chapter about a number of sleep disorders and other medical or health issues that are often associated with sleep disruption and insomnia. Although secondary insomnia can't usually be cured simply by the natural treatments described in this book, the information here can be very helpful when used as a complementary approach.

LESSER-KNOWN SLEEP DISORDERS

In recent years, researchers working with polysomnographic technology and other specialized techniques have made great strides in identifying the various conditions that interfere with normal sleep. As a result, many sleep disorders, even previously unfamiliar ones, are now readily identifiable and can often be treated successfully.

Sleep Apnea

A sleep apnea sufferer briefly stops breathing, for up to one minute at a time, hundreds of times a night, which results in very fragmented, poor-quality sleep. The National Institutes of Health reports that more than twelve million Americans suffer from this distressing and potentially serious disorder. It is an often-overlooked cause of significant sleep disruption, however, because a person with sleep apnea might not realize that he or she has difficulty breathing while sleeping.

There are three types of sleep apnea: obstructive, central, and mixed. In obstructive sleep apnea, which is by far the most prevalent, tissues in the upper airway (such as the muscles at the back of the throat) become overly relaxed during sleep and obstruct the breathing passage. In central sleep apnea, the air passages are not blocked but the brain doesn't properly signal the muscles to breathe, so the diaphragm and chest muscles stop working periodically; this occurs in people who have some type of serious neurological or other illness. Mixed apnea, a combination of the other two types, is treated the same way as obstructive apnea.

Obstructive sleep apnea is most common in men, people who are overweight, snorers, older people, and children with enlarged tonsils or adenoids. Obstructive apnea is characterized by an abnormal breathing pattern: loud snoring, pauses in breathing, and snorts or gasps as the sleeper attempts to resume normal breathing. During those pauses, oxygen in the bloodstream falls to dangerously low levels, triggering the body to gasp for breath to correct the deficit.

Although people with apnea of any type are often completely unaware that they are awakening frequently throughout the night, they may be well aware of their drowsiness and often experience daytime symptoms such as headache and difficulties concentrating. If left untreated, apnea can lead to high blood pressure, heart failure, and lung disease. If you suspect that you may have sleep apnea, consider going to a sleep disorders specialist for professional evaluation and diagnosis, which may involve spending a night in a sleep laboratory.

Excess fat in the neck compresses the airway and excess abdominal weight interferes with proper breathing, so obstructive sleep apnea in someone who is overweight can often be effectively treated with weight loss. Occasionally, surgery may be appropriate if an anatomical abnormality (an excessively fleshy soft palate or swollen tonsils, for example) is obstructing airflow to the lungs, but these surgeries are rarely 100-percent effective. Specially made dental appliances are sometimes used in treating sleep apnea to keep the air passages open.

One of the most successful treatment protocols for sleep apnea is called continuous positive airway pressure (CPAP), which utilizes a device to assist nighttime breathing. While sleeping, the person wears a mask over the nose and a steady stream of air flows through the mask to keep the airway open. Several types of CPAP devices are available; some even sense when air is needed, based on inhalation and exhalation, and can vary the level of air delivered accordingly. The biggest drawback to CPAP is patient compliance—or rather, noncompliance—as many people find the devices uncomfortable (at least initially), but those who continue using them often report significantly improved sleep and enhanced daytime energy.

If you suffer from any type of sleep apnea, it's best to not drink alcohol, especially during the evening, as alcohol depresses the breathing reflex and makes the condition worse. Because many common medications including tranquilizers, some beta-blockers, and sleep-aids also interfere with the breathing reflex, consult your doctor about any drugs you are taking and their possible alternatives. And of course, if you smoke, you should stop; smoking decreases lung capacity.

Restless Legs Syndrome

Restless legs syndrome or RLS is characterized by uncomfortable, sometimes painful sensations such as tingling or crawling feelings in the legs. The sensations are generally worse while sitting, lying down, or resting but are relieved temporarily with movement. Involuntary jerking and twitching of the legs is common in RLS, especially during sleep. Although these muscle contractions last only for a second, they occur approximately every thirty seconds, over the course of an hour or more, several times a night. The sleeper is usually unaware of the movements but sleep quality suffers.

More than 15 percent of adults are afflicted with RLS. More women than men are affected and the incidence of the syndrome increases with age. Genetics seem to play a role, as close to half of the people with RLS have a family history of the disorder. Interestingly, almost one-quarter of pregnant women suffer from RLS during pregnancy. Certain medical conditions including arthritis, varicose veins, and diabetes are associated with a higher incidence of the disorder.

Although the cause of RLS is not known, researchers suspect the involvement of neurological problems: for example, nerve impairment in the spinal cord or an imbalance in the brain's neurotransmitters (chemical messengers), especially dopamine and serotonin. A variety of lifestyle factors including smoking, caffeine, excessive alcohol intake, fatigue, and emotional stress contribute to RLS. A deficiency of iron can be the trigger. Some medications such as antidepressants, antihistamines, beta-blockers, and diuretics can also cause RLS.

Although there is no recognized cure for RLS, several simple lifestyle changes should provide relief. Supplemental iron or other nutrients may be useful (see Chapter 4 for more details). Regular moderate exercise is one of the most helpful things you can do to ease restless legs (see Chapter 10). Gentle stretching exercises such as yoga are excellent for calming the nervous system and can be done at any time during the day; but if you have RLS or leg cramps at night (see Nocturnal Leg Cramps, below), you might find it most helpful to stretch shortly before going to bed. Many people with RLS find it beneficial to take a warm bath before bed (adding 2 cups of Epsom salts and several drops of calming essential oils will enhance the relaxing effects: see Aromatherapy on page 116), whereas others get relief from cold compresses applied to the legs before bed or during an episode of restless legs. Massaging the legs and feet, especially prior to going to sleep, can be very helpful for easing RLS and ensuring a peaceful night's rest.

Nocturnal Leg Cramps

Nocturnal leg cramps, commonly referred to as charley horses, are painful muscle spasms in the calf (and sometimes in the thigh or foot) that occur one or more times throughout the night and last anywhere from several seconds to several minutes. Nocturnal leg cramps can strike anyone but are especially prevalent in adolescents, pregnant women, and the elderly.

The most common causes of nocturnal leg cramps are dehydration and an imbalance of electrolytes (dissolved trace minerals in the blood and body tissues). Electrolytes of sodium, potassium, calcium, and magnesium are critical for proper nerve and muscle function. Diuretics, diarrhea, or excessive perspiration can upset the balance of these minerals. Ensuring that your body is consistently well hydrated is essential for preventing muscle cramps in general and nocturnal cramps in particular. If you frequently suffer from any type of muscle cramps, you may not be getting enough potassium in your diet. Eating more potassium-rich foods may solve your problem or you could try taking supplemental magnesium, which has a powerful relaxing effect on the muscular and nervous systems (see Chapter 4 for more nutritional information).

Some people find relief from nocturnal leg cramps by sleeping with their feet slightly elevated on a pillow. Other tips, if you suffer from these cramps, are to avoid sleeping under heavy blankets and also to avoid pointing your toes while in bed, as toe-pointing triggers contractions in the calf muscles. If your calf does start to contract, immediately straighten your leg and flex your foot hard toward your head, then sit up and massage your calf muscle firmly. Gentle stretching exercises before bedtime also help prevent nocturnal leg cramps (see Chapter 10).

Nightmares and Night Terrors

Nightmares tend to plague children between the ages of three and eight and are considered in most cases to be part of the normal developmental process. These frightening, often vividly memorable dreams occur less frequently in adults but after a particularly traumatic event such as an accident or the death of a loved one, recurring nightmares about the event are common. Daily life stressors such as relationship problems or financial difficulties can also lead to nightmares; physical illness, fever, or certain medications are additional contributing factors.

If you are taking any medications and suffer from nightmares, consult your doctor to determine whether a drug may be affecting your sleep and causing your bad dreams. If not, consider that your nightmares may be an attempt by your subconscious mind to convey a message to you. Keeping a journal (see page 100) can be a helpful tool for remembering and decoding your dreams and many of the available books on dreams contain in-depth information about methods for understanding them. If your nightmares are frequent or particularly disturbing, you might try working with a skilled therapist to uncover and alleviate the stressors that may be at the root of your unconscious unrest.

Although nightmares and night terrors are commonly confused for each other, the two are very different. Nightmares generally occur several hours after going to sleep, during the REM stage of general bodily paralysis and active dreaming, whereas night terrors arise during stage 4, a deep, non-REM stage that takes place as early as the first hour of sleep. Night terrors are characterized by screaming, crying, or moaning, sitting bolt upright or flailing about, rapid heart rate and breathing, and sweating. An episode of night terrors resembles an intense anxiety reaction and generally lasts from a few minutes up to twenty minutes. While the sleeper's eyes may be open, he or she is actually still asleep and may have no recollection of the incident by the following day. The best approach to take with someone in the throes of a night terror is to soothe the sleeper back into normal sleep.

Factors that contribute to night terrors include being overly tired, eating a heavy meal just before bed, and taking certain medications. If you experience night terrors, check with your physician about the possible side effects of any medications you use. Antidepressants are often prescribed for recurrent night terrors; a natural alternative to pharmaceutical treatment is the herb St. John's wort (see Chapter 7). The regular practice of relaxation techniques (see Chapters 10 and 11) can promote a restful night's sleep. Mildly sedating herbs such as chamomile (see Chapter 5) and relaxing fragrant oils such as lavender (see Chapter 11) can also help you set the tone for a peaceful sleep free from nightmares and night terrors.

Seasonal Affective Disorder

Many people associate occasional gloomy feelings with occasional gloomy weather. But seasonal affective disorder, commonly referred to as SAD, is a specific form of depression related to the decrease in sunlight that occurs during the late fall and winter months. Symptoms of SAD include fatigue, oversleeping, overeating (especially sweet or starchy foods), weight gain, low energy, irritability, difficulty concentrating, and a loss of interest in previously pleasurable activities.

Researchers believe that SAD is a natural bodily response to seasonal light changes; increased darkness promotes increased melatonin secretion, which triggers the desire to sleep and affects circadian rhythms by influencing the internal biological clock (see The Gross Anatomy of Sleep on page 3). People who are susceptible to SAD experience their symptoms at approximately the same time every year and experience a full remission during the spring and summer months. Many animals slow down or hibernate during the winter but hibernation isn't generally an option for humans.

One of the most effective treatments for SAD is phototherapy or light therapy, which uses bright light to suppress the secretion of melatonin, helping to decrease the desire for excessive sleep and reduce symptoms of depression. If you suffer from a mild case of SAD, simply making the effort to spend at least thirty minutes outdoors in the sunlight each day can alleviate your symptoms. For a more severe case (or if you live in a particularly dreary climate), you'll probably need a specially made "light box" that you sit in front of for about thirty minutes a day to ensure that your retinas are exposed to adequate full-spectrum light. Antidepressant drugs are frequently prescribed for SAD; the herb St. John's wort is a natural alternative, without the negative side effects of pharmaceutical antidepressants (see Chapter 7 for more information).

Narcolepsy

Narcolepsy, an uncommon disorder of the body's sleep-regulating mechanisms, dramatically affects both sides of the sleep/wake cycle. It's best characterized, however, by the intrusion of one or more aspects of REM sleep into the waking state. The primary symptom of narcolepsy is excessive daytime sleepiness, with involuntary sleep attacks that last for thirty seconds to thirty minutes or longer. These attacks (shown in polysomnographic studies to be episodes of REM sleep) are not related to the amount of nighttime sleep obtained. They occur throughout the day and regardless of the sufferer's activity—even while working, eating, talking, or driving.

Other common symptoms of narcolepsy include cataplexy (sudden temporary muscle weakness or paralysis triggered by a strong emotion such as laughter, anger, or fear), sleep paralysis (temporary paralysis when falling asleep or awakening), and hypnagogic hallucinations (vivid mental images at the onset of sleep). The combinations and severity of narcoleptic symptoms vary greatly among individuals. Typically, the symptoms first appear in adolescence, but people with narcolepsy often go undiagnosed or misdiagnosed for years.

Although genetics and/or autoimmunity appear to play a role in this neurological disorder, the precise cause of narcolepsy is unknown and there is no cure. Stimulant drugs are used to counteract the daytime sleepiness and antidepressants to alleviate cataplexy and REM-sleep symptoms; if you have narcolepsy, you may require these prescription drugs but you can likely reduce your need for medications and support your overall health and well-being by following some of the suggestions in this book.

Narcolepsy is also controlled with behavioral therapies such as adopting a regular sleep schedule that includes scheduled daytime naps.

MEDICAL AND PHYSICAL CONDITIONS THAT DISRUPT SLEEP

A variety of disorders and conditions, both mundane and mysterious, include sleep disruption among their symptoms or effects. Some, like prostate enlargement or acid reflux, are relatively simple to identify and treat. Others are more complicated and may require a trial-and-error approach to diagnosis and treatment. Chronic fatigue syndrome and fibromyalgia, for example, share many characteristics and can be difficult to separate; they are often misdiagnosed, misunderstood, and inappropriately treated.

Chronic Fatigue Syndrome

The primary characteristic of chronic fatigue syndrome (also known as chronic fatigue immune dysfunction syndrome or CFIDS) is overwhelming exhaustion—unrelieved by a good night's sleep—that interferes with normal life activities. This debilitating condition is significantly different from the ordinary fatigue that everyone experiences after unaccustomed physical activity or a long day at work.

Because of its characteristic muscle and joint aches, sore throat, headaches, and tender lymph nodes, CFIDS is often compared to a bad case of the flu; but unlike the flu, these symptoms persist for six months or even longer. Numerous additional symptoms including irritable bowel syndrome, allergies, heart palpitations, dizziness, shortness of breath, tingling or burning sensations in the extremities, visual disturbances, ringing in the ears, and menstrual problems are associated with CFIDS. Cognitive and emotional disturbances such as depression, anxiety, and difficulties with concentration and memory frequently accompany the syndrome as well.

Many people first notice symptoms of CFIDS following a bout with a severe cold or flu, mononucleosis, bronchitis, or hepatitis. Intense, prolonged stress can also trigger the initiation of symptoms. For the majority of CFIDS sufferers, their symptoms peak fairly early in the course of the illness and then tend to come and go over time. Because the symptoms and severity vary markedly from one person to the next and because no specific laboratory test can conclusively identify CFIDS, many people with this condition may go undiagnosed.

The Centers for Disease Control estimates that approximately 500,000 people in the United States are affected by CFIDS and has established the following criteria to aid in diagnosis: unexplained fatigue not caused by ongoing exertion and not relieved by rest, which causes a significant reduction in previous levels of activity. In addition, the fatigue must be accompanied by four or more of the following symptoms that have been present for six months or longer: impaired memory or concentration, sore throat, tender lymph nodes, muscle pain, joint pain, new headaches, unrefreshing sleep, and exhaustion for at least twenty-four hours following activity. (See also Fibromyalgia, below.)

If you suspect that you are suffering from CFIDS, it's important to find an appropriate healthcare practitioner who can rule out other illnesses such as impaired thyroid function and diabetes (which share some of the same symptoms as CFIDS) and assist you in your recovery. For most people, effective treatment of chronic fatigue involves a comprehensive approach to rebuilding health, managing symptoms, and restoring energy. This generally entails making dietary and lifestyle modifications, taking specific nutritional and herbal supplements, and using supportive therapies to alleviate symptoms and promote vitality. You'll find many suggestions in this book (see Chapter 4 and Chapters 7–11) that will help you create your own healing program. Supplemental melatonin and 5-HTP, for example, are especially useful for restoring healthy sleeping patterns and for increasing levels of serotonin (see Chapter 8).

Fibromyalgia

Fibromyalgia is recognized as the second most common form of arthritis after osteoarthritis and is estimated to afflict about 2 to 4 percent of Americans. The disorder was officially defined in 1990 by the American College of Rheumatologists as the presence of widespread chronic pain for at least three months, with tenderness in at least eleven of eighteen specific points in the muscles of the arms, legs, back, and chest when moderate pressure is applied. Although fibromyalgia doesn't cause actual joint damage or deformity, as does osteoarthritis, it often seriously hinders normal functioning.

In addition to the chronic pain and tender points, common symptoms include fatigue that significantly interferes with the activities of daily life, anxiety or depression, digestive disturbances, chronic headaches, tingling sensations in the extremities, and difficulty concentrating. The majority of people who suffer from fibromyalgia also experience sleep problems including difficulty falling asleep, waking during the night or early morning hours, and not feeling rested even after sufficient sleep. It becomes a vicious cycle; sleep disruption exacerbates the symptoms of fibromyalgia and fibromyalgia disrupts sleep.

Interestingly, polysomnographic studies have shown that people with fibromyalgia don't obtain sufficient delta sleep, the stage of deep sleep when the body performs important restorative activities (see Deep Non-REM Sleep on page 5). A reduced amount of delta sleep results in a reduced output of hormones by the pituitary gland, especially growth hormone, which stimulates tissue repair, and melatonin, which regulates the body's sleep/wake cycle (see How Melatonin Works on page 84). Insufficient deep sleep also causes fatigue, morning grogginess, impaired concentration, and irritability.

Fibromyalgia symptoms can last for weeks or months, mysteriously improve or even disappear for a while, and then reappear. An accurate diagnosis depends upon providing a thorough case history to an appropriate healthcare practitioner who can exclude other conditions (such as low thyroid function) that may be causing the symptoms. Many times, symptoms first appear after a traumatic incident such as an auto accident or a sports injury or following a severe viral infection such as the flu, but no one knows for certain what causes fibromyalgia. Long-standing nutritional deficiencies, food allergies, exposure to toxic environmental chemicals, and emotional stress are all thought to play a role in the development of the illness. Whatever the triggering factor may be, many researchers believe that fibromyalgia is ultimately the result of an imbalance in serotonin or other brain chemicals that are linked to mood and sleep.

A special consideration for people suffering from fibromyalgia—and possibly for people with chronic fatigue syndrome—is the involvement of chronic inflammation in the disease process. Chemical messengers called cytokines play an essential role in regulating the immune system and are responsible for the inflammatory response that normally helps the body fight off infection. Heightened cytokine activity, however, is known to cause joint damage in rheumatoid arthritis and researchers are just beginning to understand the other types of havoc that cytokines can wreak in addition to inflammation: fever, fatigue, and achiness, which are characteristic symptoms of chronic fatigue and fibromyalgia. A study published in the July 2001 issue of *Rheumatology* reported altered production of cytokines in patients with fibromyalgia, noting that their cytokine production increased with the duration of the illness.

Conventional treatment for fibromyalgia often relies on antidepressants, tranquilizers, and sedatives for sleep, along with anti-inflammatory drugs and muscle relaxants. Natural alternatives include the herbal antidepressant St. John's wort (see Chapter 7) and various sedative herbs (see Chapters 5 and 6). Supplemental melatonin can improve sleep quality and supplemental 5-HTP stimulates the increase of serotonin levels, which aids in pain relief (see Chapter 8). As with chronic fatigue, healing from fibromyalgia and easing its symptoms involves dietary and lifestyle modifications, specific nutritional and herbal supplements, and supportive therapies (see Chapters 9–11). Dietary modifications are one of the most effective ways of suppressing inflammatory cytokines (see Chapter 4).

Gastroesophageal Reflux

Gastroesophageal reflux, known to most people as heartburn, is a familiar culprit in middle-of-the-night awakening. In this condition, the stomach contents back up into the esophagus (the tube that runs from the mouth down to the stomach) and irritate its sensitive lining. Reflux often produces a burning sensation in the chest and throat along with coughing and choking, but not everyone who suffers from acid reflux exhibits clear-cut symptoms; some people may only be aware of an acidic or bitter taste in the mouth upon waking in the morning. *Note:* Pain or tightness in the mid-chest area is another common symptom of gastroesophageal reflux and may be mistaken for a heart attack. If you experience these symptoms, it's essential to check with your doctor to rule out heart trouble.

Reflux is most often caused by a weakening of the lower esophageal sphincter (the muscular opening) at the bottom of the esophagus. Normally, as food travels down the esophagus, the sphincter relaxes, allowing food into the stomach, and then closes, keeping the food and stomach acids safely confined. But if the sphincter loses its ability to close tightly, stomach acids splash up into the esophagus. In severe cases of reflux, the esophagus can become scarred from continually being bathed in these corrosive acids.

Because lying down allows stomach contents to back up more easily, gastroesophageal reflux is more problematic at night than during the day. Nocturnal reflux can significantly disturb sleep even if the sufferer doesn't fully awaken. Many people who've experienced nighttime reflux find it beneficial to elevate the head of the bed (using bricks, for example) by about 6 inches; alternatively, you can use a special body-wedge pillow to elevate your upper body. To help protect against heartburn, don't lie down after meals and make sure not to eat within three hours of bedtime. You should also avoid anything that constricts the abdomen soon after eating, because the resulting pressure can force the stomach contents up into the esophagus; this includes bending over, wearing clothing that is too tight around the waist, or lifting heavy items.

Having large meals, eating too quickly, and drinking excessive amounts of liquid with meals are prime contributors to gastroesophageal reflux, as are certain foods and drugs (see Chapter 4). If you frequently suffer from heartburn, keeping a food/symptom diary can enable you to pinpoint the specific foods that are causing you problems. In general, it's best to avoid over-the-counter antacids. Some contain large amounts of sodium, which is contraindicated for people with high blood pressure or cardiovascular disease. Calcium antacids frequently cause rebound acid production, worsening the problem of acid reflux. Instead, try herbal antacids, which have no negative side effects (see Herbs for Better Sleep on page 51).

Benign Prostatic Hypertrophy

Benign prostatic hypertrophy or BPH is the medical term for non-cancerous enlargement of the prostate gland. This condition is a common affliction among men, affecting almost 90 percent of men by the age of eighty. One of the most pronounced symptoms of BPH is a need to get up frequently during the night to urinate—as often as five or six times. Other symptoms include a frequent need to urinate during the day and difficulty in voluntarily starting and stopping the flow of urine. The disorder generally progresses slowly over a period of months or years, with the need to urinate during the night increasing over time to several trips to the bathroom. Obviously, this disrupts normal sleep, causing fatigue and sleep deprivation.

The traditional medical approach to BPH is drugs or surgery or both. There is also a proven herbal remedy that is almost always helpful for relieving BPH symptoms: the berries of the saw palmetto, a scrubby palm native to Florida (for more details, see Benign prostatic hypertrophy on page 53). *Note:* If you suspect that you may have prostate enlargement, check with your doctor, as diagnosis and treatment of BPH should be pursued under medical supervision.

Insomnia and Medications

Most of us are familiar with medication labels that warn of possible daytime drowsiness but it is less widely recognized that many commonly used medications also disturb sleep to a considerable degree. Some of these drugs delay the onset of sleep, some cause awakening in the middle of the night, and some cause early morning awakening. Many prescription drugs, including those used to treat asthma and allergies, contain stimulants that interfere with sleep. Medications for high blood pressure and heart disease (such as the frequently prescribed beta-blockers) cause insomnia at night and drowsiness during the day. Diuretics (drugs that increase the elimination of salts and fluids from the body) stimulate urination, resulting in nighttime awakenings. Dehydration caused by diuretics can also contribute to fatigue.

Over-the-counter medications frequently disturb sleep because their formulas may include powerful stimulants. Nasal decongestants, for example, often contain the stimulant ephedrine or pseudoephedrine, and some pain-relief medications, including many for headaches and menstrual cramps, contain caffeine. An adverse reaction to a prescription or over-the-counter medication may occur immediately or a person may suddenly develop intolerance to a drug after using it for years. If you suffer from insomnia and are taking any medications for any other condition or illness, inform your doctor. Most likely, an alternative medication can be found that doesn't have the side effect of insomnia.

Menopause and Insomnia

During menopause, many women experience some type of sleep disturbance as a result of hormonal changes. The conventional medical approach to menopausal symptoms from hot flashes, night sweats, heart palpitations, and insomnia to irritability, anxiety, and depression is hormone replacement therapy (HRT). Synthetic hormones, however, often have unpleasant side effects such as headaches, breast soreness, nausea, and acne. More dangerously, conventional HRT puts a woman at greater risk for high blood pressure, gallbladder disease, blood clots, and breast cancer. (Natural hormones that have much less risk of side effects are available by prescription through a naturopathic physician or a doctor who practices a holistic approach.) Fortunately, many women find relief from menopausal symptoms by making dietary changes, getting regular exercise and plenty

Adrenal Gland Depletion and Menopause

As discussed in Chapter 2, the adrenal glands play a central role in the body's reaction to physical and emotional stressors. When you perceive a situation as stressful, your adrenal glands secrete hormones, including adrenaline and corticosteroids, that increase heart rate and breathing, raise blood pressure, and trigger the release of glucose into the bloodstream for quick energy. This powerful response has worked well to ensure our survival as a species by providing the capacity to either fight or run away from a dangerous situation. But under the unrelenting stress that is typical of modern life, overworked adrenal glands can become exhausted by continually operating as though a condition of extreme danger exists.

These glands play another very important role for women entering menopause. When the ovaries slow down and eventually cease their production of hormones, the adrenal glands normally take over that function; although the amount of estrogen they produce is small compared to what the ovaries once generated, they should be able to make enough to ease the transition through menopause. Unfortunately, by the time many women reach menopause, their adrenal glands are not up to the task of making sufficient hormones to maintain health and vitality. Common symptoms of adrenal depletion include fatigue, depression, insomnia, hypoglycemia, poor concentration, and lowered immunity.

With care, however, it's possible to rejuvenate the adrenal system. Any steps that you can take to reduce stress in your life will help ease the demands on your adrenals. Rest and sufficient sleep are essential—albeit difficult for someone with insomnia to achieve easily! To support adrenal health, the most significant dietary change you can make is to restore a healthy balance of potassium and sodium by eating at least seven servings of fresh vegetables and fruits daily and cutting down on sodium. The B-complex vitamins, vitamin C, magnesium, and zinc are especially important. Siberian ginseng (*Eleutherococcus senticosus*) is an excellent herb for helping to rebuild adrenal health. Avoid caffeine and refined sugars, which provide a temporary boost of energy but further deplete the adrenals. (See Chapter 4 for more details on nutritional support in menopause.)

of rest, and using nutritional supplements and herbs to help regulate their hormone levels.

At midlife, the foods that a woman chooses to eat (and those that she avoids) have a significant effect on how her body adapts to the changes of menopause. Certain foods have a profound effect on hormone levels, particularly foods that are rich in phytoestrogens, which are plant compounds with weak estrogenic properties (they're approximately fifty times weaker than human estrogen). These compounds are able to attach to receptor sites in the body that are normally occupied by estrogen and can help balance a woman's declining estrogen levels. Certain supplements and herbs are also valuable allies for women in menopause. (See the inset "Adrenal Gland Depletion and Menopause" on page 38 and also Chapter 4 for information on nutritional and herbal approaches to menopausal symptoms.)

4

Diet and Nutrition for Restful Sleep and Optimal Energy

I t may seem obvious that eating healthfully immediately affects your energy level and mood and that your dietary choices are a critical factor in preventing or developing degenerative diseases such as heart disease, cancer, and diabetes. It may surprise you, however, to realize that the foods you eat—and the foods you avoid—have a profound influence on how well you sleep. Researchers are discovering almost daily the remarkable benefits of health-enhancing compounds found in many natural, unprocessed foods, as well as in nutritional supplements and herbs. Think of it this way: each time you eat, you have the opportunity to improve your overall well-being and that includes your sleep/wake cycle. It's important to pay attention to how particular foods affect you and to minimize intake of anything that taxes your body. In this chapter, you'll learn about what to eat and drink for better sleep.

EATING WELL FOR LIVING WELL—AND SLEEPING WELL

Eating well means providing your body with all of the proteins, carbohydrates, fats, vitamins, minerals, and calories it needs for daily energy as well as for nighttime maintenance and repair. Ideally, the foods you eat should be delicious and satisfying and they should nourish you with optimum levels of nutrients. A simple way to accomplish this is to make your diet "nutrient dense" by eating a variety of fresh foods (see the inset "Basics of a Nutrient-Dense Diet"). Eating well means drinking well too. To stay well-hydrated and maintain healthy organ function, we need about 2 quarts of water daily. Not drinking enough fluids causes dehydration and enables toxins to accumulate, both of which can cause fatigue.

The Principles of a Healthful Diet

Although a diet high in complex carbohydrates and low in fat has been popularized for years as the most healthful way of eating, many people find that a diet consisting primarily of carbohydrates—even healthful complex carbohydrates—increases insulin levels and causes fatigue, weight gain, and hormonal imbalances. Nutrition research now indicates that increasing intake of protein and healthful fats while reducing carbohydrate intake (especially simple carbohydrates and sugars) balances blood sugar and hormones, resulting in a more stable energy level. Although no single diet is perfect for everyone, the following basic principles will help just about everyone build a nutritional foundation for good health. Take the time to find a way of eating that makes you feel healthy and energetic. Pay attention to how foods affect you and don't be afraid to experiment. To feel your best, you need to discover the diet and the eating schedule that best support your particular body, genetic makeup, and lifestyle.

Base Your Diet on Whole, Unrefined, Nutrient-Dense Foods

Fresh, natural, minimally processed foods are the richest in nutrients,

---

Basics of a Nutrient-Dense Diet

- Fresh vegetables: five or more servings daily (emphasize nutrient-rich dark leafy green and deep yellow-orange vegetables)
- Fresh fruit: two to three servings daily (berries and citrus fruits are particularly good sources of phytonutrients)
- Lean protein: two to three servings daily (eat cold-water fish such as salmon and sardines often—they are rich in important omega-3 fatty acids)
- Complex carbohydrates: two or more servings daily (such as whole grains, legumes, yams, and winter squash)
- Healthful fats: approximately 30 percent of your daily diet (extra-virgin olive oil, raw nuts and seeds, avocados)
- Calcium-rich foods: two to three servings daily (low-fat dairy products, dark leafy greens, sardines, sesame seeds, almonds)
- Pure water: four to six glasses daily

including the trace minerals and other compounds that are critical for optimal health. Make fresh vegetables and fruits, lean proteins, whole grains, low-fat dairy products, and healthful fats the center of your diet. Minimize consumption of over-processed foods such as pasta, white rice, and products made with refined flour and sugar; use these only occasionally instead of relying on them as daily fare.

Eat a Wide Variety of Foods

Most people get into dietary ruts, eating only a handful of foods. Broadening your food choices provides you with a wider array of vitamins, minerals, antioxidants (compounds that neutralize cell-damaging free radicals), essential fatty acids (fats that cannot be produced by our bodies), and phytonutrients (health-protective compounds found in plants) that support optimal health. In addition, eating a variety of foods decreases the possibility of creating food sensitivities that can arise when the same few foods are eaten day after day.

Eat an Abundance of Fresh Vegetables and Fruits

Fresh vegetables and fruits provide a wide range of antioxidants and phytonutrients that help prevent disease and slow the aging process. Try to eat at least seven, preferably nine, servings daily. A serving is $1/2$ cup or one medium-sized piece of fruit, $1/2$ cup of vegetable, or 1 cup of leafy greens. Choose vegetables and fruits with the deepest colors, as they tend to have the most nutrients.

Eat High-Quality Proteins

Protein is essential for rebuilding healthy tissue and it helps stabilize blood sugar levels as well. Eat three servings daily, choosing from lean proteins including fish, poultry, eggs, dried cooked beans, legumes, and soy foods such as tempeh and tofu.

Eat Plenty of High-Fiber Foods

Fiber speeds up the movement of wastes through the intestinal tract, helping to cleanse the body of toxic chemicals such as pesticides. Fiber also aids in the elimination of excess estrogen and cholesterol. To obtain the health benefits of different fibers, eat a variety of whole grains, legumes, vegetables, and fruits.

Eat Beneficial Fats

Some fats are harmful to the body (see Subtle Sleep Disruptors on page 55). Healthful fats, however, are actually protective against cancer, heart disease, and other degenerative diseases. These "good" fats are found in extra-virgin olive oil, nuts, seeds, avocados, and cold-water fish. Fat also helps balance blood sugar levels by slowing the release of stored glucose into the bloodstream. In addition, fat is necessary for the body's production of prostaglandins, hormonelike substances that are essential for hormone balance and proper immune function.

Eat Calcium-Rich Foods

Calcium maintains bone strength and keeps your nervous system functioning properly. To obtain 1,000–1,200 milligrams of calcium daily, include a wide variety of calcium-rich foods such as almonds, dark leafy greens, dairy products, legumes, oranges, sesame seeds, tofu, and sardines in your diet and take calcium supplements if necessary (see Nutritional Supplements for Better Sleep on page 48).

Drink Plenty of Water

About half of your daily fluid requirement (2 quarts) is provided in the foods that you eat, especially if you consume plenty of vegetables and fruits. Pure spring water or filtered water is the best option for supplying the rest of the fluids that your body needs. Get into the habit of drinking four to six glasses of water daily, preferably between meals.

Avoid Foods Grown, Treated, or Processed with Chemicals

We all have residues of pesticides and other chemicals stored in our body tissues. Such poisons enter our food supply in a variety of ways; pesticides and other agricultural chemicals are applied to crops, hormones and antibiotics are fed to the animals raised for the meat and dairy industries, and a huge assortment of chemicals is added to foods during processing. These toxins are a primary cause of degenerative diseases and premature aging. Whenever possible, buy organically grown and processed foods.

Avoid Excess Sugar

Sugars, including sucrose, glucose, maltose, dextrose, corn syrup, honey (fructose), molasses, and maple syrup, cause fluctuations in blood sugar levels that are stressful on the body and are a primary cause of fatigue. Ideally, eat sugar as it occurs naturally in whole foods like fresh fruits and sweet vegetables such as carrot, winter squash, and sweet potato. To help curb your sugar cravings and stabilize your blood sugar levels, make sure that your diet includes adequate amounts of protein and healthful fat.

Avoid Caffeine

Caffeine is a powerful drug that stresses your nervous system and contributes to insomnia and anxiety (see Caffeine and Insomnia on page 56). It overstimulates the adrenal glands and places the body in a state of chronic stress, resulting in fatigue after the initial stimulant effect wears off. Coffee, black tea, green tea, chocolate, colas and other soft drinks, and many over-the-counter drugs such as stimulants, cold remedies, and pain medications contain caffeine—check labels.

Dietary Suggestions for Better Sleep

There are many foods that promote sound, restful sleep in general and some foods that are specifically helpful for particular sleep problems. Timing matters too; when you eat also has an effect on how well you sleep. If possible, try to make breakfast and lunch the most substantial meals of your day and keep your dinner fairly light. Because digestion is an active process, eating a heavy meal at night can interfere with good-quality sleep. Examples of light, nutritious dinners are a large salad with grilled fish, a bowl of soup, whole-grain bread, and a salad, or a stir-fry of poultry or tempeh with vegetables and brown rice. Just as important as not overeating, however, is ensuring that you do eat enough to maintain a stable blood sugar level. Fluctuations in blood sugar, which cause daytime fatigue, are also a common cause of middle-of-the-night awakenings.

If you eat dinner three or more hours prior to bedtime or if you tend to awaken during the night, you might find it helpful to have a small snack about thirty minutes before bed. Eating a healthful, balanced snack that combines protein with a small amount of "good" fat and complex carbohydrates will help keep your blood sugar level consistent throughout the night. Try a few whole-grain crackers with peanut butter, an apple and a small handful of walnuts, or a piece of fruit and a slice of cheese.

A snack before bedtime can also boost brain levels of the neurotransmitter serotonin, which acts as a natural sedative. Because serotonin is made by the body from the amino acid tryptophan, you can increase your serotonin levels by eating foods that are rich in tryptophan (see

Chapter 8); good sources include avocados, bananas, cheese, chicken, cottage cheese, fish, legumes, milk, nuts, and turkey. Eating a small portion of complex carbohydrates at the same time enhances the absorption of tryptophan.

Another important consideration in normalizing or boosting serotonin levels is to make sure your diet includes plenty of the building blocks that form serotonin receptors in the brain. These receptors are made primarily from omega-3 fatty acids, the beneficial fats found in cold-water fish such as salmon, mackerel, herring, and sardines. Walnuts and flaxseeds are good vegetarian sources of these essential fatty acids.

Eating to Bolster Stress Resistance

As discussed in Chapters 2 and 9, adopting healthful ways of managing stress is one of the most important things you can do to get a better night's sleep. But no matter how good you get at defusing stress, it's not possible to avoid it altogether; you can however, reduce its impact nutritionally. Fresh vegetables and fruits, for example, supply potassium, a critical nutrient for proper adrenal gland function (see the inset "Foods for Adrenal Support" on page 46). The surge in adrenaline that occurs as part of the physiological stress response increases the metabolism of available protein, fats, and carbohydrates, which gives your body the energy it needs to deal with the crisis. A nutrient-rich diet is therefore essential for helping your body cope with stressful situations.

To bolster your stress resistance nutritionally, follow this chapter's guidelines for a health-enhancing diet and take special care to avoid food stressors such as caffeine, alcohol, and refined carbohydrates. Caffeine, for example, is a major factor in triggering feelings of anxiety. Even small amounts can cause restlessness, heart palpitations, headaches, insomnia, and nervousness, so you should consider eliminating all sources of caffeine if you are troubled by any of these conditions. Alcohol, though it is often used as a relaxant, can also affect the endocrine and nervous systems in ways that intensify anxiety, agitation, and depression. Overeating, particularly of sweets and refined carbohydrates, is another favorite coping mechanism for many people but is itself stressful to the body (see Food Stressors to Avoid or Eliminate on page 55). Instead, choose complex carbohydrates, found abundantly in whole grains, vegetables, legumes, fruits, seeds, and nuts. These healthful foods help stabilize blood sugar levels and supply steady energy to your body and brain.

Foods for Adrenal Support

To support adrenal health, make sure to eat foods that are rich in vitamins C, B_5, and B_6, magnesium, and zinc (see also Nutritional Supplements for Better Sleep on page 48).

● Many fruits and vegetables, including broccoli, grapefruit, oranges, red peppers, and strawberries, contain vitamin C.

● Pantothenic acid (vitamin B_5) is found in avocados, chicken, eggs, mushrooms, salmon, and yogurt.

● Bananas, lentils, tempeh, trout, and tuna are good sources of vitamin B_6.

● Plentiful amounts of zinc are found in black beans, pumpkin and sesame seeds, mussels, and oysters.

● Almonds, corn, halibut, tofu, and peas are rich in magnesium.

Dietary Tips for Specific Sleep Problems

In addition to this chapter's general dietary guidelines for improved health and sleep overall, the following suggestions can be helpful for relieving specific sleep problems related to jet lag, leg cramps, restless legs, chronic fatigue, fibromyalgia, reflux, and menopause.

- **Jet lag.** To lessen the impact of traveling across time zones, make sure to drink plenty of fluids while flying to keep your body well-hydrated but avoid alcoholic beverages, which cause dehydration and intensify the symptoms of jet lag. In addition, eat small, frequent meals built around protein, healthful fats, and complex carbohydrates to keep your blood sugar levels balanced and prevent travel fatigue. (See also Herbal Tips for Specific Sleep Problems on page 52.)

- **Nocturnal leg cramps.** Make it a habit to drink at least six to eight glasses of water daily to keep your body well-hydrated. If you are exercising heavily, you might want to try an electrolyte-replacement drink to quickly restore normal mineral balance. These are often sold as "sports drinks," but you can make your own without artificial colors or other additives (see the inset "Natural Electrolyte-Replacement Drink" on page 47). Electrolytes of potassium and magnesium are particularly helpful for preventing nocturnal leg cramps and are easily obtained through a healthful diet. Bananas, cooked dried beans, oranges, potatoes, spinach, and tomatoes are excellent sources of potassium. Magnesium is found in foods such as whole grains, legumes, nuts, seeds, and leafy greens. (See also Supplement Tips for Specific Sleep Problems on page 50.)

- **Chronic fatigue and fibromyalgia.** There are numerous dietary strategies for preventing or reducing the inflammation that is implicated in both of these syndromes. To provide your body with omega-3 fatty acids, which help in calming inflammation, eat a serving of cold-water fish such as salmon or sardines at least three times a week and include a tablespoon of flaxseeds or flaxseed oil in your daily diet. Eating lots of fresh vegetables

> ## Natural Electrolyte-Replacement Drink
>
> Combine 1 quart of water with 2 tablespoons of honey and $\frac{1}{2}$ teaspoon of sea salt. Sip approximately 1 cup of this beverage before exercising and another after exercising. Drink enough so that you are well hydrated but not so much that you feel bloated and uncomfortable.

and fruits every day provides vitamin C, vitamin K, and other anti-inflammatory phytochemicals as well. (See also Supplement Tips for Specific Sleep Problems on page 50.)

Avoid the over-consumption of omega-6 fatty acids (found in polyunsaturated fats) and saturated fats (found primarily in red meat and full-fat dairy products). Strictly avoid hydrogenated fats and trans-fatty acids (found in shortening, margarine, and many processed chips, crackers, and baked goods). These "bad" fats stimulate the production of compounds called cytokines that instigate the immune system's inflammatory response. In addition, avoid sugar and refined carbohydrates, which contribute to inflammation by triggering spikes in insulin production.

- **Gastroesophageal reflux.** To help prevent reflux, eat smaller meals, chew food thoroughly, sip only small amounts of liquids with meals (drink most of your liquids between meals), and make mealtimes peaceful and stress-free. Remember that coffee, tea, chocolate, alcohol, carbonated beverages, fatty foods, smoking, and aspirin are primary culprits in heartburn. Some people are also sensitive to mint and to acidic forms of vitamin C such as those made from ascorbic acid. (See also Herbal Tips for Specific Sleep Problems on page 52.)

- **Menopause.** Eat frequent small meals that include plenty of high-quality proteins such as chicken, fish, and eggs and avoid simple carbohydrates such as sugar and white-flour products. This helps stabilize blood sugar levels and prevent the fatigue that besets many women during menopause. Support your adrenal glands, which play an important role in maintaining your vitality, by cutting down on sodium and eating at least seven servings per day of potassium-rich vegetables and fruits (see the inset "Foods for Adrenal Support" on page 46).

Because phytoestrogens can help regulate and supplement estrogen levels in menopause, it's a good idea to eat several servings daily of foods such as whole grains, nuts, flaxseeds, and legumes, which are rich in these helpful compounds. Soybeans and soy products are of special value, because soy is an excellent source of particular phytoestrogens called isoflavones. In fact, researchers believe that high consumption of soy isoflavones is the reason that Japanese women have an easier time during menopause. Isoflavones are also available as supplements but it's best to include isoflavones in your diet in the form of soy foods instead. Although research indicates that a daily serving of soy ($^1/_2$ cup of tofu or tempeh or 1 cup of soy milk) is protective for your health, no one is certain of the effects of supplemental isoflavones. Some researchers have expressed concern that high doses of concentrated isoflavones may contribute to estrogen-dependent cancers such as certain forms of breast cancer.

Omega-3 fatty acids are also important during the menopausal years to aid in balancing hormones. Good sources of omega-3 fats are cold-water fish (such as salmon and sardines), walnuts, and flaxseed. To ensure that you're getting sufficient amounts of these beneficial fats, eat one or two servings of these foods daily. (See also Supplement Tips for Specific Sleep Problems on page 50.)

Nutritional Supplements for Better Sleep

Even if you consistently eat a balanced diet, it's difficult to obtain optimal amounts of every nutrient through food, especially if stress or any other chronic problem has exhausted your body's stores of an important vitamin or mineral. Don't rely on supplements alone to build up your health but do include them as part of a comprehensive approach to creating energy, vitality, and longevity.

Start by choosing a high-quality, high-potency, multivitamin-mineral supplement that provides a wide range of the basic micronutrients including vitamins A, B-complex, C, D, E, and K, carotenoids, calcium, magnesium, selenium, zinc, and other trace minerals (see the Appendix). *Note:* If you are a man or a post-menopausal women, do not take a supplement that contains iron unless advised to do so by your doctor, because iron can accumulate to dangerous levels in the body and is implicated in certain forms of cancer and heart disease.

For best results with nutritional supplements, take capsules, which are more easily broken down in the digestive tract than tablets are, and take them with meals. Food enhances supplement absorption and lessens the possibility of stomach upset.

The following micronutrients are especially vital in any nutritional approach to improving sleep. If your multivitamin-mineral supplement doesn't supply the dosages recommended below, take additional supplements as needed.

B-Complex Vitamins

Not only does stress deplete the body of B-complex vitamins but a deficiency in these can also contribute to some sleep disorders including restless legs syndrome and menopausal sleep disruption. Be sure that your supplements provide 25–50 milligrams per day of B_1, B_2, B_3, B_5, and B_6 plus 400 micrograms of folic acid. Don't take B-complex vitamins late in the evening, because they can be stimulating—this stimulating effect, however, can be used to your advantage during the day, for naturally boosting your energy level.

Calcium

Because calcium calms the nervous system and has a mild sedative effect, it is generally helpful for all types of sleep-related disorders. Take 800 milligrams of calcium daily; or if you do not eat many calcium-rich foods, take 1,200 milligrams daily. Calcium citrate is the most easily absorbed form of this mineral. For best assimilation, divide the total daily amount you're taking into two doses and have them with meals.

Magnesium

Magnesium, being a muscle and nervous system relaxant, helps relieve sleep-related muscle cramping. Many factors deplete magnesium, including emotional and physical stress and alcohol. Take 400–600 milligrams of magnesium daily in the form of magnesium citrate, malate, aspartate, gluconate, or lactate. *Note:* Taking more than 600 milligrams of magnesium daily can cause diarrhea.

Chromium

Chromium plays a key role in blood sugar metabolism and is helpful if you have blood sugar fluctuations that awaken you during the night. To help stabilize your blood sugar level, take 200 micrograms of chromium daily. *Note:* Do not exceed the recommended dosage of chromium without consulting your doctor.

Supplement Tips for Specific Sleep Problems

Particular vitamin and mineral supplements are especially helpful for restless legs, nocturnal leg cramps, chronic fatigue and fibromyalgia, and the sleep disruption associated with menopause.

- **Restless legs syndrome.** Some studies have shown that people with restless legs syndrome are deficient in iron; other studies point to an impairment in the way that certain parts of the brain utilize iron, causing a deficiency of the neurotransmitter dopamine, which is involved in muscle movement. Supplemental iron may help with restless legs but you should never take iron supplements without first confirming with your doctor, through a simple blood test, that your level of iron is low. The body is not able to easily rid itself of excess iron and the mineral can rapidly accumulate to dangerous amounts in body tissues, causing irreversible damage to the heart and other organs.

  As folic acid deficiency is one suspected cause of RLS, try supplementing your diet with folic acid by taking 400 micrograms daily along with 25–50 milligrams of B-complex vitamins; these are often sufficiently supplied by a high-potency multivitamin-mineral formula. (See also B-Complex Vitamins on page 49.) Other supplements that can be helpful for alleviating RLS symptoms are vitamin E taken in the form of d-alpha tocopherol at a daily dose of 400–800 international units and magnesium at 400–600 milligrams daily. (See also Magnesium on page 49.)

- **Nocturnal leg cramps.** If you suffer from nocturnal leg cramps, you may benefit from taking a magnesium supplement just before bed. To provide adequate levels of magnesium, take 400–600 milligrams daily in an easily absorbable form such as magnesium citrate, aspartate, gluconate, or lactate. In addition to being a relaxant, magnesium can also act as a laxative agent and sometimes causes loose stools, so decrease your dosage if necessary. (See also Magnesium on page 49.)

- **Chronic fatigue and fibromyalgia.** Essential vitamins for curbing inflammation include the B-complex vitamins (25–50 milligrams daily), vitamin C (500 milligrams daily), and vitamin E (400–800 international units daily). Another very useful anti-inflammatory supplement is 240 milligrams daily of gamma-linolenic acid or GLA, often taken in the form of evening primrose oil or borage seed oil. (See also B-Complex Vitamins on page 49.)

- **Menopause.** Take a high-potency multivitamin-mineral supplement, along with additional supplements if necessary, to obtain 250–500 milligrams of vitamin C, 50–100 milligrams of the B-complex vitamins, 400 milligrams of magnesium, and 25 milligrams of zinc daily; supporting adrenal health in this way enhances vitality and helps the body adjust more easily to the hormonal fluctuations of menopause. And taking calcium (1,200 milligrams daily), in addition to strengthening bones, is beneficial for menopause-related insomnia. (See also B-Complex Vitamins on page 49; Magnesium on page 49; and Calcium on page 49.)

Herbs for Better Sleep

Certain herbs are very well known for providing symptomatic relief of emotional and physical tension and for promoting relaxation or even sleep. Gentle sedative herbs such as chamomile or lemon balm may be sufficient to ease mild tension and can be used as daily beverage teas. The simple act of brewing and sipping a cup of tea is a relaxing ritual and provides a welcome respite in the midst of a busy day. More powerful stress-relieving herbs that are helpful during periods of intense anxiety include kava and valerian. (See Chapters 5 and 6 for details on using these herbs for stress and insomnia.) A longer-term approach to the psychophysiological relief of stress and anxiety, however, is based on strengthening the endocrine and nervous systems.

The adrenal glands, an integral part of the endocrine system, are key players in the body's response to stress (see The Impact of Stress on page 20). Chronic stress taxes adrenal function and can actually shrink the glands. Typical signs of adrenal exhaustion include feelings of fatigue, stress, and anxiety. Herbs that bolster the endocrine system can play a key role in helping the body adjust to stress. Siberian ginseng (*Eleutherococcus senticosus*), for example, is an excellent herbal tonic that can be taken over the long term to improve the body's response to stressful situations, build resistance to stress and anxiety, and enhance resilience to physical and emotional stressors. By strengthening the adrenal glands, this herb moderates the detrimental effects of stress on the body. It helps restore vitality, increase energy, and improve mental and physical performance (see the inset "Herbal Energizers" on page 57). *Note:* Although Siberian ginseng is very safe, taking higher-than-recommended doses can potentially cause insomnia, anxiety, and irritability.

Remember, though, that herbs are not in themselves a cure for stress and anxiety. Herbal sedatives are useful for short-term relief but trying to use herbs to cover up or suppress the root of these distressing emotions will not be effective in the long term; underlying causes of stress, anxiety, and depression must be addressed. Your psyche is speaking to you through your body's physical symptoms and your symptoms will likely worsen until you give them the attention they demand.

Herbal Tips for Specific Sleep Problems

The following herbs can provide relief for symptoms of jet lag, gastroesophageal reflux, prostate enlargement, and menopause that wreak havoc with sleep.

- **Jet lag.** Russian cosmonauts were given Siberian ginseng to help them adjust their biological rhythms while in space. Studies have proven that this herb is helpful against more ordinary jet lag as well. If you want to use Siberian ginseng solely to relieve and possibly prevent the symptoms of jet lag, start taking it one week prior to travel and continue taking it for one week following your flight: $^1/_2$–1 teaspoon of liquid extract or 1,000 milligrams of powdered herb in capsules twice daily. If you're taking a standardized extract, follow the manufacturer's instructions or take 200–400 milligrams daily.

  Passionflower is an herb that can be used to alleviate jet lag by promoting nighttime relaxation. Take 1 teaspoon of liquid passionflower extract in a small amount of warm water one hour before bedtime and follow this with a second dose fifteen minutes before actually going to bed. (See Chapter 5 for more information about using passionflower.)

- **Gastroesophageal reflux.** A cup of tea brewed from chamomile or ginger (*Zingiber officinale*) after meals can calm the digestive tract and prevent sleep-disturbing reflux; both of these herbs have soothing anti-inflammatory properties. (See Chapter 5 for more information about using chamomile.)

For recurrent problems with acid reflux, try deglycyrrhizinated licorice root (*Glycyrrhiza glabra*), conveniently abbreviated as DGL. DGL is an excellent anti-inflammatory agent and helps decrease the production of excess stomach acid. To help ease the symptoms of acid reflux, take $\frac{1}{4}$ teaspoon of powdered DGL with water, fifteen minutes before meals, up to four times a day.

- **Benign prostatic hypertrophy.** Native Americans used the berries of the saw palmetto (*Serenoa repens*) to treat genitourinary problems including prostate irritation. Compounds isolated from saw palmetto berries are known to dramatically inhibit the production of dihydrotestosterone, the male hormone responsible for benign prostatic hypertrophy (BPH). European studies show that saw palmetto decreases BPH symptoms including difficulty in urinating, frequent urination, and pain, usually within three months or less (see the inset "Saw Palmetto versus Conventional BPH Treatment" below). This herb is bitter and soapy tasting—it's not something you want to drink as a tea. To obtain adequate amounts of the identified active ingredients, you should take an extract of saw palmetto berries that is standardized to contain 85 to 95 percent fatty acids and sterols, at a dosage of 160 milligrams twice a day.

Saw Palmetto versus Conventional BPH Treatment

The standard pharmaceutical treatment for BPH is a prescription drug called Proscar, which benefits only about half of the men who try it, takes about six months to have an effect, and costs approximately $75 a month. By contrast, saw palmetto extract relieves symptoms in almost 90 percent of the men who try it in just four to six weeks and is one-fourth the cost of Proscar. The side effects of many of the conventional drug therapies and surgical procedures for benign prostate enlargement include possible impotence. Saw palmetto, on the other hand, has no harmful side effects and has traditionally been used as a sexual rejuvenator.

- **Menopause.** Siberian ginseng has been studied extensively in the former Soviet Union, where it is greatly valued for its ability to help the body adapt to physical and emotional stress. To obtain the full benefits of Siberian ginseng for adrenal support in menopause, the herb must be used for two to three months. Take 1 gram of powdered root, $^1/_2$–1 teaspoon of fluid extract, or 100–200 milligrams of an extract standardized for eleutherosides, twice daily. Siberian ginseng can be used indefinitely. *Note:* Although Siberian ginseng is very safe, taking higher-than-recommended doses can cause insomnia, anxiety, and irritability.

  Of the various plants that have been used for centuries to ease menopausal difficulties, black cohosh (*Actaea racemosa* or *Cimicifuga racemosa*) is especially helpful for women suffering from estrogen imbalance. Black cohosh has been shown in at least twenty clinical studies to be as effective as synthetic estrogen for relieving menopausal symptoms such as hot flashes, night sweats, heart palpitations, irritability, and depression. In one multicenter German study of 629 women, 80 percent of the participants taking the herb reported improvement within six to eight weeks. Although relief is not immediate, black cohosh is far safer than synthetic hormones and has no toxicity or harmful side effects. Clinical studies have generally used black cohosh extracts standardized for their content of triterpenes, the compounds considered to be the active ingredients. The typical study dosage of black

---

Hot Flash Tea

Motherwort, a wonderful herb for menopausal women, has relaxing properties and helps calm the heart palpitations that often accompany hot flashes. Aniseed, which adds a pleasant sweetness to the tea, is a source of phytoestrogens that help balance the declining estrogen levels that trigger hot flashes. The aromatic oil giving garden sage its characteristic scent is a powerful astringent that reduces perspiration by up to 50 percent.

Pour 1 cup of boiling water over 2 teaspoons each of garden sage and motherwort and 1 teaspoon of aniseed. Cover and let steep for fifteen minutes. Strain the tea, sweeten if desired, and drink 1 cup before bedtime; or, drink it during the night if you awaken with a hot flash.

cohosh amounts to 4 milligrams of triterpenes daily. Black cohosh can also be taken as one 500–600 milligram capsule of the powdered herb three times a day or approximately $\frac{1}{2}$ teaspoon of a liquid extract twice daily; if you're taking a standardized extract, follow the recommendations on the manufacturer's label.

A tea brewed from motherwort (*Leonurus cardiaca*), aniseed (*Pimpinella anisum*), and garden sage (*Salvia officinalis*) can also provide relief from sleep-disruptive hot flashes (see the inset "Hot Flash Tea" on page 54).

FOOD STRESSORS TO AVOID OR ELIMINATE

In addition to the foods you eat and the supplements and herbs you take, a few other diet-related considerations influence how well you sleep.

Obviously, to avoid disrupting your night's sleep, you should avoid eating or drinking anything that you've found to trigger indigestion or gastroesophageal reflux. Fatty foods, coffee, tea, chocolate, and alcohol are common causes of heartburn and some people also have difficulties with spicy foods.

Subtle Sleep Disrupters

Eating sugar is a primary cause of fatigue. Sweets and other refined carbohydrates have an initial soothing and sedating effect on the nervous system but they trigger a rapid increase in blood sugar that is quickly followed by a sharp drop. These fluctuations in blood sugar level exacerbate stress and anxiety and are the cause of many physical symptoms including headaches, irritability, daytime dips in energy, and nighttime sleep disturbance.

It's also best to avoid drinking alcohol. Although alcohol has an initial relaxing effect that can help you fall asleep, it typically causes awakening several hours later. This interrupts sleep's natural progression into the deeper, restorative stages and interferes with the normal, healthful cycles of delta and REM sleep (see The Stages of Sleep on page 4).

Food intolerances or sensitivities—which are more difficult to diagnose than actual food allergies—also contribute to sleep disruption for some people. Food sensitivities can cause chronic health problems such as tension, restlessness, fatigue, mood swings, and insomnia. The most common triggers of food sensitivity problems are chocolate, corn, dairy products, eggs, soy, and wheat. If you suspect that food sensitivities are a problem for you, you might consider keeping a food/symptom journal, in which you keep track of everything you eat and any symptoms you notice for at least one month. With this type of record-keeping, you should be able to discern whether there is a connection between your sleep problem and the foods you are eating.

Caffeine and Insomnia

Caffeine is a common culprit in insomnia and should always be considered a possible contributor to any sleep problem. As a stimulant and a diuretic, not only does caffeine delay falling asleep at night but it can also lead to middle-of-the-night awakenings. People vary in their susceptibility to the effects of caffeine; some may be able to easily metabolize a cup or two of coffee daily whereas others are so sensitive to caffeine that they can't tolerate even the trace amounts found in decaffeinated coffee or tea. It's also not unusual to become less caffeine-tolerant with age.

Because caffeine is an accepted and widely used drug in our society, it's easy to overlook the fact that it is, in fact, a powerful stimulant. One of the most addictive aspects of caffeine is that it provides an immediate boost of energy and alertness; many people rely on it to jump-start the day or to help them through an afternoon slump. Giving up caffeine is challenging for almost everyone—but if you suffer from any type of sleep disturbance, kicking caffeine is essential. Along with trouble sleeping, caffeine is linked to numerous health problems: nervousness, anxiety, gastrointestinal upset, increased blood pressure, heart rhythm disturbances, and symptoms of premenstrual syndrome, among many others.

Breaking a caffeine habit almost always incurs withdrawal symptoms, most commonly headaches. You can take plain aspirin for these headaches (avoid caffeinated pain-relievers such as Excedrin). If you prefer an herbal alternative, valerian (see Chapter 6) has a strong sedative effect and can help ease the pain, but don't expect it to be as effective as aspirin. For caffeine-withdrawal headaches, take $1/2$–1 teaspoon of valerian liquid extract up to four times a day as needed.

If you are patient and persistent, you can minimize the discomfort of withdrawal by gradually reducing your intake of coffee and other caffeinated substances. For example, cut back on your morning coffee from two cups to one or brew a mixture of half regular coffee and half decaffeinated. If you experience withdrawal symptoms, stay at that level of caffeine intake for three days or until the symptoms disappear, then gradually cut back a bit more, continuing until you have completely eliminated caffeine.

Herbal Energizers

If you've been depending on caffeine for energy and are looking for a healthful alternative, consider taking an herbal energy tonic such as Siberian ginseng (*Eleutherococcus senticosus*). Unlike caffeine and similar stimulants, Siberian ginseng builds energy slowly over a period of time and decreases your need for a quick fix. Take 1 gram of powdered root, $1/2$–1 teaspoon of liquid extract, or 100–200 milligrams of an extract standardized for eleutherosides, twice a day. You should see a noticeable increase in your energy level after about three months.

Green tea (*Camellia sinensis*) contains a compound called l-theanine that promotes feelings of relaxed alertness, providing an immediate natural energy boost. Green tea is rich in other phytochemicals that have numerous health-protective benefits as well. (And fortunately, l-theanine is found in decaffeinated green tea.)

If you decide to give up caffeine "cold turkey," it will likely take about three days before withdrawal symptoms subside and you're feeling back to normal. Do yourself a favor by planning your withdrawal over a long weekend, when you can rest and treat yourself gently. Sleep as much as possible; take warm, soothing baths with ten drops of lavender essential oil to help you relax; and get a massage to relieve muscle tension. For distraction, watch videos, read a good book, or do whatever else appeals to you to take your mind off of your discomfort. Exercise can also help by increasing energy and stimulating the body's detoxification.

Although coffee is a primary source of caffeine, numerous other beverages, foods, and even medicines also contain significant amounts of the drug: black and green teas, cola drinks, chocolate, coffee-flavored ice creams and candies, and some over-the-counter and prescription drugs, especially pain relievers, cold medicines, weight-loss formulas, and menstrual cramp medications (check the labels). In eliminating caffeinated beverages from your diet, it's important to find satisfying substitutes; to discover your favorites, experiment with the wide variety of herbal teas, grain coffees, and other available alternatives (see the inset "Herbal Energizers" above).

5

Mild Herbs for Stress and Insomnia: Chamomile, Hops, Lemon Balm, and Passionflower

Certain herbs have been valued for centuries for their calming and relaxing properties and have long been used to treat sleep disorders. In Europe, where herbs are regarded as an accepted form of conventional medicine, organizations such as the European Scientific Co-operative on Phytotherapy (ESCOP) now issue suggestions for the modern therapeutic uses of herbs.

Herbs are available in a variety of forms including capsules, concentrated liquid extracts (these may be alcohol based or glycerin based), and dried in bulk for making teas. Some herbs are also offered as standardized extracts, which are formulated to contain a specific amount of the ingredient(s) thought to be responsible for the herb's healing properties. (Unless otherwise specified, all herbal dosage recommendations given in this book are for nonstandardized products.)

In this chapter, you'll learn about chamomile, hops, lemon balm, and passionflower, which are the mildest of the herbal sleep-aids. They can be used as often as needed for difficulty falling asleep or staying asleep. Although they are gentle, these relaxing herbs are also effective; however, if you don't notice a significant difference in your ability to sleep after a few times of using them, then consult the next chapter for more powerful herbal sedatives.

CHAMOMILE

One of the most popular herbs throughout history, chamomile is beloved for its applelike scent and flavor. Two varieties of chamomile are used by herbalists: *Matricaria chamomilla*, the annual German variety that grows to

3 feet tall, and *Anthemis nobilis,* a low-growing perennial called Roman or English chamomile. Both of these plants have feathery leaves and tiny dai-sylike flowers with yellow centers and white petals and both species con-tain the same essential oil that gives chamomile its healing properties. German chamomile has a more pleasant flavor, though, and is the variety primarily used as a medicinal herb.

Because of its appealing flavor, chamomile is perhaps best known as a beverage tea. It also has soothing properties when used externally and is a frequent ingredient in skin- and hair-care products. But while chamomile is gentle enough for infants and children, it is powerful enough to be an effective herbal treatment for anxiety and insomnia.

Medicinal Uses of Chamomile

Chamomile was used by the ancient Egyptians to relieve fevers and by the early Greeks and Romans and the Ayurvedic healers of ancient India to treat headaches as well as kidney, liver, and urinary tract problems. In Europe, chamomile has been used for centuries for digestive problems, insomnia, menstrual cramps, and pain relief. Early British and German immigrants introduced both varieties of chamomile to North America.

Scientific Support for Chamomile

Thousands of years of use have established chamomile as a healing herb but there hasn't been much research to verify the medicinal properties of the plant. Scientists have made a start, however, by identifying a number of therapeutic compounds in chamomile. Fragrant essential oils in the flow-ers, including bisabolol, bisabololoxides A and B, and azulenes, are anti-inflammatory and antispasmodic (relieving muscle spasms or cramps). Flavonoid compounds including apigenin and luteolin have also been found to play an important role in chamomile's healing properties. For example, laboratory findings indicate that apigenin may bind to certain receptors in the brain (the same ones that benzodiazepines do) to pro-mote a mild sedative effect and help alleviate anxiety.

In a 1995 German study, an extract of chamomile was found to effec-tively relieve anxiety in mice. Another study on mice found that cham-omile acted as a mild nervous system depressant, producing drowsiness and relaxation. Although these investigations were conducted with labo-ratory animals and not human participants, their results corroborate the traditional use of chamomile as a mild sedative. It's noteworthy that, even with a relative lack of supporting scientific research, chamomile is listed as an official drug in the pharmacopoeias of twenty-six countries including Germany, France, and the United Kingdom.

How to Use Chamomile

The simple, satisfying act of brewing a hot cup of chamomile tea can become a soothing evening ritual that helps set the stage for a peaceful night's sleep. Pour 1 cup of boiling water over 2 teaspoons of dried chamomile flowers; cover and steep for ten minutes, then strain the tea; drink it thirty minutes before bedtime. If anxiety and emotional stress are bothering you, you might consider drinking an additional 2–3 cups of chamomile tea throughout the day. If you prefer the convenience of a liquid extract, take $1/2$ teaspoon of extract diluted in a small amount of warm water one to three times a day.

Chamomile also makes a soothing and relaxing pre-bedtime bath. Add 6 tablespoons of dried chamomile flowers to 1 quart of water and bring to a boil; cover, remove from heat, and steep for twenty minutes; strain the "tea" and add it to a bathtub of comfortably warm water; then soak yourself in the herb-infused bathwater for fifteen minutes.

Cautions for Chamomile

Chamomile is generally regarded as an extremely safe and gentle herb and side effects from its use are rare. As with any medicinal herb, however, it's a good idea to note the following precautions.

- Using excessive amounts of chamomile can cause stomach upset and nausea.

- If you have a severe allergy to ragweed (species of *Ambrosia*), it's probably best to avoid chamomile, which is one of its botanical relatives. There have been some reports of allergic reactions to chamomile, primarily the Roman variety. These reactions, however, are rare, as only five cases of chamomile allergy have been documented; the relationship between ragweed allergy and chamomile is so far unsubstantiated.

- If you take prescription blood-thinning drugs such as warfarin, you should check with your physician before using medicinal amounts of chamomile. Chamomile contains natural compounds that can potentially act as blood thinners; mixing prescription and herbal blood thinners may intensify their effects.

HOPS

The characteristic bitter flavor of beer as we know it comes from the pleasantly bitter flavor of hops, which are the strobiles or conelike fruits of the climbing hop vine (*Humulus lupulus*). Sometime around the ninth century, German beermakers began putting hops in their brews to add flavor and as a natural preservative. By the fourteenth century, almost all European breweries followed suit. Along with this contribution to beer making, hops also has a long history of medicinal use. Early hop growers noticed that workers who harvested the golden strobiles in the fall tended to fall asleep in the fields, which triggered interest in using the herb as a sedative.

Medicinal Uses of Hops

Hops was a common ingredient in many patented nineteenth-century herbal tonics and was listed as a sedative in the United States Pharmacopoeia from 1831 until 1916. Herbalists today continue to recommend hops as a sedative and tranquilizer. Because the herb also has antispasmodic and muscle-relaxant properties, hops can be helpful for muscle tension that interferes with sleep. In evaluating the research on hops, ESCOP indicates it for treating tenseness, restlessness, and sleep disturbances.

Scientific Support for Hops

There hasn't been much research into the medicinal benefits of hops. Researchers do know, however, that ripe hop strobiles are rich in lupulin, a yellow powder containing the essential oil that is thought to be responsible for the herb's healing properties. More than 100 different compounds have been found in the essential oil of hops. One of these compounds, 2-methyl-3-butene-2-ol, has been found to produce sedative effects on the nervous system. Although fresh hop strobiles contain only trace amounts of the chemical, its concentration increases to significant amounts when the fruits are dried. This is one case where the dried, aged herb is much more powerful than the fresh herb.

How to Use Hops

Hops make a bitter but not unpleasant-tasting tea. Pour 1 cup of boiling water over 1–2 teaspoons of dried hop strobiles; cover and steep for ten minutes; then strain the tea, sweeten if desired, and drink it thirty minutes before bedtime. If you prefer, you can use a concentrated liquid extract of hops. Take $1/2$ teaspoon of extract diluted in a small amount of warm water thirty minutes before bed.

Hops also makes an effective sedative bath. Add 6 tablespoons of dried hop strobiles to $1^1/2$ quarts of boiling water; cover, remove from heat, and steep for twenty minutes; strain the "tea" and add it to a warm bath; then soak yourself in the herb-infused bathwater for fifteen minutes or longer, as desired.

Cautions for Hops

Hops is generally regarded as an extremely safe and gentle herb and side effects from its use are rare. As with any medicinal herb, however, it's a good idea to take note of the following precautions.

- Hop strobiles are rich in phytoestrogens, which give the plant estrogen-like properties. If you have had estrogen-dependent breast or uterine cancer, check with your doctor before using hops.

- Because of the high content of phytoestrogens in hops, women who are pregnant should not use hops in medicinal amounts.

- If you are taking prescription sedatives, check with your doctor before using hops, because combining prescription and herbal sedatives may intensify their effects.

LEMON BALM

Also called melissa (after its Latin name, *Melissa officinalis*), lemon balm is a vigorous perennial in the mint family and is native to southern Europe. The bright green leaves, which contain the herb's medicinal compounds, have a lemony aroma when crushed; a tea made from the plant has a mild lemon flavor. So well-regarded was this herb for nervous complaints that the famous seventeenth-century English herbalist Nicholas Culpepper wrote of it, *"Balm causeth the mind and heart to become merry, and driveth away all troublesome cares and thoughts arising from melancholy. . . ."*

Medicinal Uses of Lemon Balm

In the tenth century, lemon balm was a favorite of Arab physicians, who recommended it for anxiety and nervousness. Medieval Europeans took note and "melissa water" became a popular sedative—the emperor Charlemagne even ordered that the herb be grown in every medicinal garden so there would be an abundant supply. Herbalists in the Middle Ages prescribed lemon balm for insomnia, headaches, nervous stomach, anxiety, and depression. Today, herbalists still recommend lemon balm for insomnia, anxiety, and stress, as well as for wounds and viral infections, and also as a digestive aid. Germany's Commission E, a panel of herbal experts that helped establish guidelines for herbal usage, recommends lemon balm for treating insomnia.

Scientific Support for Lemon Balm

Researchers conducting studies with animals have discovered several compounds in lemon balm that have sedative properties, primarily a group of chemicals called terpenes. These and other compounds are found in the fragrant essential oil that gives the leaves their characteristic scent and flavor. The sedative effects of lemon balm also hold true for humans. In a double-blind study of twenty people comparing the effects of the herb to those of a placebo, the general consensus was that lemon balm increased calmness and reduced alertness.

In a German study of ninety-eight people, lemon balm combined with valerian (see Chapter 6 for more information on valerian) was found to improve sleep quality as compared to a placebo. Another study showed that the same herbal combination formula was as effective as the pharmaceutical tranquilizer Halcion but without the negative side effects such as morning grogginess.

How to Use Lemon Balm

To brew a tea from lemon balm, pour 1 cup of boiling water over 2 teaspoons of dried leaf (or 2 tablespoons of fresh leaves); cover, steep for fifteen minutes, and strain. For insomnia, drink 1 cup of lemon balm tea thirty minutes before bed. For general stress and anxiety, drink up to 3 cups throughout the day. If you prefer to use a concentrated liquid extract, take $1/_2$–1 teaspoon of extract, diluted in a small amount of warm water, up to three times a day.

Cautions for Lemon Balm

Lemon balm is a safe and gentle sedative herb that is appropriate for mild insomnia. Note the following precautions when using lemon balm.

• To prevent excessive sedation, consult your physician before using medicinal amounts of lemon balm if you are taking prescription sedatives, because combining prescription and herbal sedatives can intensify their effects.

- In animal studies, lemon balm has been found to depress thyroid activity by inhibiting thyroid-stimulating hormone. If you suffer from hypothyroidism (low thyroid function), you should not use medicinal amounts of lemon balm without first consulting your healthcare practitioner.

PASSIONFLOWER

Passionflower (*Passiflora incarnata*) is a native tropical American vine with scented, 3-inch purple and white flowers that bloom in May and are followed by sweet yellow fruits. The flowers and leaves are the medicinal part of this beautiful, exotic-looking plant, which can climb up to 30 feet in one season. The Incas used passionflower as a tonic tea and the herb was brought to Europe in the late 1500s, where its pleasant flavor made it a favorite.

Medicinal Uses of Passionflower

Passionflower is primarily valued for its mild sedative properties. Early colonists found the Native Americans of the Gulf Coast using local passionflower as a tea for calming anxiety. In the mid-1800s, the Eclectic physicians (a group of doctors who emphasized the use of natural treatments) viewed passionflower as an important remedy for insomnia, restlessness, menstrual discomfort, and epilepsy, among other maladies. From 1916 to 1936, passionflower was listed as a sedative in the *National Formulary*, an official reference guide for pharmacists in the United States.

Herbalists today recommend passionflower as a sedative and mild tranquilizer. In Europe, passionflower is included in many natural formulas. It's not addictive and doesn't require a prescription. ESCOP indicates the use of passionflower for tension, restlessness, and irritability with difficulty in falling asleep.

Scientific Support for Passionflower

Research has identified tranquilizing compounds in passionflower including passiflorine, a substance with chemical similarities to the powerful sedative morphine. Interestingly, passionflower also contains stimulating compounds but researchers have found that the complex interaction of the chemicals in the herb results in a mild tranquilizing effect overall.

Animal studies have shown that passionflower has a definite sedative effect and clinical studies have shown that it acts the same way in humans. In a French study, researchers gave either an herbal formula containing passionflower or a placebo to ninety-one people suffering from anxiety; after twenty-eight days, the participants given the herbal formula reported a significant decrease in feelings of anxiety. Another four-week double-blind study of thirty-six people suffering from anxiety disorder compared passionflower to the prescription sedative oxazepam. Although oxazepam took effect more quickly, passionflower demonstrated equal effectiveness at relieving anxiety symptoms by the end of the trial. The researchers also noted that passionflower did not cause the side effects (such as impaired job performance) that are typical of oxazepam.

How to Use Passionflower

Passionflower makes a pleasant-tasting tea. Pour 1 cup of boiling water over 1 teaspoon of dried passionflower leaves; cover and steep for ten to fifteen minutes; strain the tea and sweeten if desired. For insomnia, drink 1 cup of passionflower tea thirty minutes before bed. For general anxiety and restlessness, drink up to 3 cups throughout the day. If you prefer, you can use passionflower as a concentrated liquid extract. Take $1/4$–1 teaspoon of extract, diluted in a small amount of warm water, up to three times a day.

Cautions for Passionflower

Passionflower is considered safe in the amounts that are generally recommended. However, the following cautions should be observed.

- Pregnant women should not use medicinal amounts of passionflower, because certain compounds in the herb (harmala alkaloids) are uterine stimulants. Although passionflower has not been associated with miscarriage, it's wise to choose another herbal relaxant such as chamomile if you are pregnant.

- If you are taking prescription sedatives, check with your healthcare practitioner before using medicinal amounts of passionflower, because combining prescription and herbal sedatives may magnify their tranquilizing effects.

6

More Powerful Herbs for Stress and Insomnia: Valerian and Kava

S ometimes more powerful herbal sleep-aids are necessary, especially for overcoming chronic sleep disorders. Temporarily taking herbal sedatives can help reset your disrupted sleep patterns while you are making the necessary lifestyle changes that support restful sleep.

The two herbs you'll find in this chapter, valerian and kava, are among the most potent natural sedatives in the plant kingdom. For the most part, they are safe to use and in general are much safer than pharmaceutical sedatives. If you are currently taking any prescription drugs for insomnia, consult your healthcare practitioner for advice in making the transition to herbal sleep-aids. If you choose to use kava, read this chapter carefully and note the contraindications. Because of current concerns about the possible toxicity of kava for certain individuals, it's best to work with a qualified herbal practitioner when using this herb.

VALERIAN

Native to Europe and parts of northern Asia, valerian (*Valeriana officinalis*) was brought by early colonists to North America, where it now grows wild in much of the eastern United States and Canada. This tall perennial has attractive fernlike foliage with clusters of tiny pale-pink flowers in the spring. Valerian was known to ancient Greek and Roman physicians as *phu,* referring to the medicinal root's pungent, musky odor. (Cats also love the aromatic root, which affects them in much the same way as catnip.)

Medicinal Uses of Valerian

Valerian has been recognized for more than 1,000 years for easing nervous tension, muscle spasms, anxiety, and insomnia. The noted German herbalist Abbess Hildegard of Bingen recommended valerian as a sleep-aid in the twelfth century. In 1820, valerian was included as a tranquilizer in the *United States Pharmacopoeia*. It also appeared in the *National Formulary*, the pharmacist's guide, until 1946. With the advent of synthetic pharmaceutical sedatives in the 1940s, the use of valerian declined in the United States but its popularity in Europe continued.

Research has shown that valerian shortens the length of time that it takes to get to sleep, reduces the frequency of nighttime awakenings, decreases nervous tension and anxiety, and improves overall sleep quality. As a result of numerous studies, valerian was approved as a sleep-aid by Germany's Commission E in 1985. The herb is also approved as an over-the-counter sedative in France, Italy, Switzerland, and Belgium. Today, valerian is one of the most commonly prescribed herbal remedies for insomnia. It's also recommended for anxiety, tension, and stress-related headaches and digestive disturbances.

Scientific Support for Valerian

Even though valerian clearly exhibits powerful tranquilizing properties, researchers don't know exactly how the herb creates its sedative effects. Numerous theories abound and more than one may ultimately prove to be correct. Scientists have discovered that one or more compounds in valerian appear to bind to benzodiazepine receptors in the brain, similarly to the action of sedative drugs such as Valium. On the other hand, another compound in valerian may also block the brain's uptake of the neurotransmitter serotonin in the same way that Prozac and other antidepressant drugs act. Some of the compounds in valerian that are under investigation by scientists include valerenic acid, valepotriates, and the volatile essential oils that give the plant its characteristic odor.

A number of studies, mostly European, have confirmed valerian's usefulness as a sleep-aid. Five placebo-controlled experiments and several large multicenter studies of more than 11,000 people have shown valerian to be an effective sedative and to improve sleep quality. In one German study, researchers gave a valerian extract or a placebo one hour before bedtime to 121 people suffering from insomnia. The majority of participants who were given the herbal extract experienced significant improvement in sleep quality. In another German study, sixty-eight adults with chronic insomnia received either a combination of valerian and lemon balm extract (see Chapter 5 for more about lemon balm) or a placebo. Those who took the herbal combination fell asleep more quickly, slept longer, and reported significantly greater feelings of well-being.

Other clinical studies have reported similar positive results comparing valerian to prescription drugs in the benzodiazepine class. In a twenty-eight-day double-blind trial of seventy-five people with insomnia, valerian was shown to be as effective a sedative as oxazepam. Another double-blind study of forty-six patients with insomnia showed that an herbal combination of valerian and hops was as effective as the sedative bromazepam. Although valerian appears to have similar tranquilizing effects on the nervous system, it is much milder and safer than benzodiazepines, which have serious side effects including impaired coordination, dizziness, mood disturbances, and possible addiction (see Chapter 12). Valerian is not addictive, nor does discontinuation of valerian cause the withdrawal symptoms of insomnia, nausea, and agitation that are associated with benzodiazepines.

How to Use Valerian

Valerian can be made into a tea, although the pungent flavor and odor discourage many people from drinking it. To make valerian tea, pour 1 cup of boiling water over 1 teaspoon of dried chopped root; cover and steep for ten minutes; strain the tea and sweeten if desired. For help getting to sleep at night, drink 1 cup of this tea thirty minutes before bedtime.

Many people prefer to use a concentrated liquid extract or capsules of powdered valerian root for insomnia. Take $1/2$–1 teaspoon of extract or 300–500 milligrams of powdered root in capsules thirty minutes before bedtime. It may take up to four weeks to stabilize sleep patterns; studies have shown that the effectiveness of valerian increases over time. This is the opposite result usually obtained with many conventional sleep medications, which tend to diminish in effectiveness with continued use.

Cautions for Valerian

Valerian is safe when used as directed but it's a good idea to take note of the following precautions.

- Occasionally, valerian may cause stomach upset. If this occurs, take the herb along with a snack such as a couple of crackers.

- As with any powerful sedative, valerian should not be used within a couple of hours of driving or operating machinery.

- When used as recommended, valerian does not cause the morning grogginess typical with prescription sedatives. Taking very large amounts of the herb, however, may cause grogginess.

- Although valerian is not dangerous when combined with alcoholic beverages (as are prescription sedatives), be aware that the herb may intensify the effects of alcohol.

- If you are taking prescription sedatives, check with your doctor before taking valerian, because combining prescription and herbal sedatives can magnify their effects.

- Interestingly, anecdotal evidence suggests that valerian can cause stimulation in some people instead of sedation. Although this is unlikely to happen, switch to another sedative herb if you experience this paradoxical effect.

KAVA

Kava (*Piper methysticum*), sometimes called kava kava, has been cultivated for centuries in Polynesia. A large perennial shrub in the pepper family, kava has attractive heart-shaped leaves; the root of the plant, however, is the part used medicinally, ceremonially, and socially. The Latin name for kava (*methysticum*) is derived from the Greek word *methys* meaning "intoxicated," which describes the herb's effects if taken in large amounts.

Kava has been used for hundreds of years as a ceremonial herb in the Pacific Islands. When village chieftains and elders gather for meetings, grated or pounded kava root is mixed with coconut milk or water in a coconut shell and each person drinks a couple of bowls of the kava beverage. The herb has a calming effect and promotes a sociable atmosphere. In an eighteenth-century voyage to the South Pacific, British explorer James Cook and his crew were invited to participate in kava ceremonies and were the first to report the mildly intoxicating effects of kava to the Western world. Kava is also used less formally by the islanders in much the same way that alcohol is used in the West—as a relaxant in social situations.

Medicinal Uses of Kava

Kava is primarily used for treating anxiety, stress, and insomnia. The herb has a mild tranquilizing effect similar to Valium. Kava, however, is not addictive, and in normal doses it elicits feelings of general well-being instead of sedation. Kava has become increasingly popular in the West for its ability to immediately relieve stress. Unlike prescription tranquilizers, kava calms the mind without affecting the ability to concentrate. It also acts as a gentle muscle relaxant and pain-reliever and has been prescribed for treating chronic disorders such as fibromyalgia (see Fibromyalgia on page 33). In larger doses, the herb acts as a sedative and is helpful for sleep disorders.

Kava was long believed to be very safe and, on the basis of several double-blind studies, was approved by Germany's Commission E in 1990 for the treatment of anxiety, stress, and agitation. Recently, however, kava has been associated with rare but potentially fatal cases of liver damage (see Cautions for Kava on page 72 and the inset "Is It Safe to Use Kava?" on page 71).

Scientific Support for Kava

Initial laboratory studies of kava root in Germany in the fifties and sixties culminated in the identification and isolation of compounds called kavalactones, which were determined to have sedative, pain-relieving, and muscle-relaxing effects. Scientists are not certain, though, exactly how kava exerts its sedative action. Some researchers have found that kava affects receptors for the neurotransmitter gamma-aminobutyric acid (GABA) in the brain, thereby promoting feelings of relaxation. Other studies have shown that kava acts on the brain's limbic system, a part of the brain that influences the emotions. Kava has also been found to block the uptake of noradrenalin by certain other parts of the brain; noradrenalin is a hormone that triggers the physiological stress response (see The Impact of Stress on page 20).

Numerous studies have demonstrated the calming effects of kava on anxiety and stress. In a well-designed placebo-controlled German study of 100 people suffering from various forms of anxiety, the participants who were given 300 milligrams of kava extract daily showed significantly less anxiety after two months, reporting a reduction in anxiety symptoms such as restlessness, nervousness, heart palpitations, stomach upset, dizziness, and chest pain. In a 1996 study, fifty-eight people suffering from general anxiety received either 100 milligrams of kava three times a day or a placebo and their anxiety was measured with standard clinical tests. After only one week, the participants taking kava reported a lessening of symptoms such as nervousness and tension; improvements in the kava group continued for the four weeks of the study, with no side effects.

Is It Safe to Use Kava?

Although kava has been clearly implicated in at least a few cases of liver toxicity, no scientific studies to date have proven that kava causes liver damage, so the question of the herb's possible toxicity remains unanswered. For example, the reported problems could have resulted from interaction between kava and other medications; those who became ill could have had a preexisting liver disease such as hepatitis; or, a high intake of alcohol could have been a factor in some cases.

It's worth noting that kava has been used for centuries in the South Pacific without reports of harmful side effects. In addition, research studies conducted on kava have shown only minor side effects (such as gastrointestinal upset) in a very small percentage of people. By contrast, it's interesting to note that thousands of toxic reactions and deaths are caused every year by common over-the-counter aspirin and Tylenol (acetaminophen). In fact, according to a report in the 2002 *Annals of Internal Medicine,* acetaminophen overdose is the leading cause of acute liver failure in the United States.

There's no question that kava is a valuable herbal medicine; further studies are needed to determine what risk, if any, is actually associated with the herb. To be safe, follow these precautions suggested by the American Botanical Council.

- Do not take kava if you have a history of liver problems without first consulting your physician.

- Do not take kava if you are taking any drugs (including over-the-counter drugs) that have known adverse effects on the liver.

- Do not take kava if you regularly consume alcohol.

- Do not take kava daily for more than four weeks without the advice of a qualified healthcare practitioner.

- Stop using kava immediately and consult your physician if symptoms of liver toxicity occur: for example, brown urine, yellowing of the eyes, nausea or vomiting, light-colored stools, unusual fatigue or weakness, stomach or abdominal pain, or loss of appetite.

Kava has also been found to be as effective as standard prescription anti-anxiety drugs. In a six-month double-blind study of 174 people, kava was found to relieve anxiety as successfully as the benzodiazepines oxazepam and bromazepam.

How to Use Kava

Kava is available in a wide variety of forms including powdered extracts, liquid extracts, and capsules. *Note:* Do not exceed recommended doses of kava and do not take the herb for more than four weeks without consulting a qualified health practitioner (see also Cautions for Kava, below).

Kava is often sold as a standardized extract with the amount of kavalactones per dose listed on the label. For the treatment of anxiety with standardized kava, the usual recommendation is to take 40–70 milligrams of kavalactones three times per day. When standardized kava is taken specifically as a sedative for insomnia, a dose of approximately 180–210 milligrams of kavalactones thirty minutes before bedtime is appropriate.

If you choose to use nonstandardized kava products, the general recommended dosage for anxiety is one 500-milligram capsule up to three times a day or fifteen to thirty drops of liquid extract up to three times a day. For insomnia, the usual recommendation is two capsules or $1/2$ teaspoon of liquid extract thirty minutes before bedtime.

Cautions for Kava

A growing number of reports in recent years have raised serious concerns about the safety of consuming kava. In several cases, even at normal dosages, kava has apparently caused severe liver damage (see the inset "Is It Safe to Use Kava?" on page 71). In light of these concerns about kava's potential toxicity to the liver, it's best to consult a qualified herbalist or a healthcare practitioner familiar with herbs before using kava, especially if you plan to take it more than occasionally.

- Kava should not be taken with prescription sedatives, because combining prescription and herbal sedatives may intensify their sedative effects.

- Kava may cause gastrointestinal upset. To prevent this, take the herb with a meal or a snack.

7

An Herb for Sleep Problems Associated with Mood Disorders: St. John's Wort

Depression and anxiety are often implicated in chronic sleep disorders. If you tell your physician that you're having trouble sleeping, you'll most likely be given a prescription for a pharmaceutical antidepressant or a sedative. These commonly prescribed drugs may offer short-term relief but they often have unpleasant side effects and can be dangerously addictive. Drugs also do nothing to address the underlying causes of emotional unrest.

Many times, herbs can provide the extra physiological support that can help bring the body and mind back into balance, without dangerous side effects, and without the risk of addiction. Of all of the antidepressant herbs, St. John's wort is the most effective for helping to alleviate mild to moderate depression and anxiety. By helping to calm the nervous system, St. John's wort works on a deep level to relieve sleep disorders related to depression and anxiety. In this chapter, you'll learn about how St. John's wort works and the most effective ways to use it.

ST. JOHN'S WORT

St. John's wort (*Hypericum perforatum*) is a perennial weedy plant that is native to Europe and was introduced to America by early colonists. Its showy midsummer display of bright yellow star-shaped flowers is a common sight along roadsides and in sunny fields. Ancient Europeans believed that St. John's wort drove away evil spirits. The plant has long been used medicinally to treat a variety of maladies including nerve injuries, inflammation, sciatica, ulcers, burns, and depression.

St. John's wort plays a prominent role in the herbal medicine of modern Europe, where doctors frequently prescribe the herb for treating depression, anxiety, and insomnia. It's clearly the treatment of choice for depressive disorders in Germany, where physicians prescribe St. John's wort extracts twenty times more often than they do Prozac, a prescription antidepressant widely used in the United States.

St. John's Wort, Depression, Anxiety, and Sleep Problems

People suffering from depressive disorders typically have an imbalance of specific brain chemicals known as neurotransmitters. This chemical imbalance manifests in a variety of symptoms: physically, as changes in sleep, appetite, and energy; emotionally, as a sense of hopelessness or irritability or as a lack of interest in work, socializing, or hobbies; and mentally, as difficulty concentrating or making decisions. St. John's wort has proven helpful for alleviating all of these symptoms. As a result, the herb is highly regarded as a natural treatment for mild to moderate depression.

Trying St. John's wort as an alternative to conventional antidepressants makes sense. Pharmaceutical antidepressants have numerous side effects including dry mouth, nausea, fatigue, headache, gastrointestinal distress, sleep disturbances, and impaired sexual functioning. In contrast, St. John's wort carries little risk of side effects and those that are reported tend to be minor (such as stomach upset). The herb also costs far less than antidepressant drugs and does not require a prescription.

Antidepressants are frequently prescribed for treating chronic fatigue syndrome, fibromyalgia, and SAD, all of which involve significant sleep problems (see Chapter 3). But these drugs—especially tricyclic antidepressants and MAO inhibitors—are actually known to reduce sleep quality by interfering with REM sleep (see The Stages of Sleep on page 4). St. John's wort, on the other hand, promotes restful sleep overall and appears to enhance REM sleep in particular, offering an effective natural alternative for treating such sleep-related conditions as well as depression.

If you are currently taking prescription medication for a depressive disorder, do not begin taking St. John's wort without consulting your doctor, as combining St. John's wort and standard antidepressants can cause unwanted side effects. Never discontinue antidepressants without talking with your doctor first. Many people have switched from antidepressant drugs to St. John's wort but you should only do so under medical supervision (see Cautions for St. John's Wort on page 80).

Anxiety often plays a prominent role in depressive disorders, manifesting as feelings of restlessness and irritability as well as insomnia. Other common symptoms of anxiety include muscle tension, digestive disturbances, and heart palpitations. A certain level of anxiety is a normal reaction to specific conditions—for example, most people feel anxious when faced with a dangerous situation—but constant or chronic anxiety affects quality of life and can become debilitating.

Physicians frequently prescribe benzodiazepine medications such as Valium and Xanax for treating anxiety and the sleep problems associated with it (see Common Drugs for Sleep Problems on page 123). These drugs have numerous side effects including lethargy, drowsiness, mental impairment, and a high potential for addiction. Taking benzodiazepines can also trigger depression. A much safer approach to anxiety reduction and sleep improvement is to follow the lifestyle suggestions in this book, making sure to avoid all stimulants such as caffeine (see Caffeine and Insomnia on page 56). St. John's wort has been found to be as helpful as prescription medications in easing chronic anxiety but without the harmful side effects; it should be considered in conjunction with those lifestyle suggestions.

How St. John's Wort Works

The primary compounds in St. John's wort include flavonoids, hyperforin, hypericin, pseudohypericin, polycyclic phenols, kaempferol, luteolin, and biapigenin; scientists are still working to determine the active ingredient(s). Hypericin was originally thought to be the most significant constituent but more recent findings point to hyperforin as the ingredient responsible for the herb's mood-elevating effects and possibly for its effects on sleep. Many St. John's wort products are currently standardized to contain specific amounts of hypericin and hyperforin.

Although many clinical studies have proven the effectiveness of St. John's wort in relieving depression, scientists like to have a clear picture of exactly how an herb affects the body and brain. More investigations are underway to identify the active ingredients in St. John's wort and to figure out their precise modes of action. The theories are fairly complex, as it appears that St. John's wort may operate in somewhat roundabout ways to alleviate depressive symptoms.

People who are depressed often have low brain levels of serotonin, which is a neurotransmitter that aids communication between nerve cells and also acts as one of the body's natural "feel-good" chemicals. Some research indicates that St. John's wort inhibits the rate at which brain cells reabsorb serotonin, in a similar way to the action of some antidepressant drugs (see the inset "St. John's Wort: Not an MAOI" below). Another theory about the beneficial effect of St. John's wort is that it seems to reduce levels of interleukin-6, a protein that plays a role in communication between cells both within and outside of the immune system. Increased levels of interleukin-6 appear to stimulate a rise in cortisol and other adrenal hormones, which are biological markers for depression. It may be that St. John's wort helps relieve depression by inhibiting interleukin-6 and thereby decreasing cortisol levels.

Scientific Support for St. John's Wort

In a forty-two-day study, German physicians gave seventy-two depressed patients 900 milligrams daily of standardized St. John's wort extract or a placebo. Patients' scores on the Hamilton Depression Scale (a standard test to measure depression) declined by 55 percent for those taking St. John's wort but only dropped by 28 percent for those taking the placebo. Patients who received St. John's wort also showed improvement in symptoms after only one week of taking the herb, with significant peaks in positive response after twenty-eight and forty-two days. No side effects were reported.

A number of other studies support the use of St. John's wort for both depression and anxiety; as a beneficial "side effect," the herb has been

St. John's Wort: Not an MAOI

At one time, St. John's wort was thought to act in a similar way to monoamine oxidase inhibitors (MAOIs), an older class of antidepressant drugs. For this reason, people taking the herb were cautioned to avoid foods high in the amino acid tyramine (such as red wine, aged cheese, and chocolate) because the interaction of tyramine-rich foods with MAOIs can cause blood pressure levels to become dangerously elevated, producing symptoms including headaches, palpitations, and nausea. More recent research, however, has not confirmed St. John's wort to be an MAOI. Instead, it is now thought to act like a more recently developed class of antidepressant drugs, the selective serotonin-reuptake inhibitors (SSRIs) that increase levels of serotonin in the brain.

found to improve sleep patterns as well. As a result, St. John's wort is also being used to treat seasonal affective disorder (SAD) and fibromyalgia (see Chapter 3).

St. John's Wort Compared to Prescription Antidepressants

In a six-week German study, 240 patients suffering from mild to moderate depression were given either 500 milligrams of standardized St. John's wort extract daily or Prozac. Although assessment with the Hamilton Depression Scale showed an approximately 12 percent decline in depressive symptoms for both groups of patients at the end of the six-week trial, assessment with the Clinical Global Impression Scale showed that St. John's wort was significantly more effective in relieving the patients' depression than Prozac. Only six people taking St. John's wort complained of side effects and these were limited to gastrointestinal symptoms, whereas thirty-four people taking Prozac reported side effects including gastrointestinal problems, vomiting, agitation, dizziness, and erectile dysfunction.

In a seven-week study conducted by Ronald Brenner, M.D. and associates of the St. John's Episcopal Hospital in Far Rockaway, New York, thirty depressed patients received either 600–900 milligrams of a standardized extract of St. John's wort daily or the prescription antidepressant Zoloft. Depression was measured using the Hamilton Depression Scale and the Clinical Global Impression Scale. Brenner reported significant improvements in the group taking St. John's wort within two weeks. After six weeks, depressive symptoms were reduced by an average of 47 percent in the patients taking St. John's wort and 40 percent in those taking Zoloft. Two people taking St. John's wort reported dizziness and two people taking Zoloft reported nausea or headache.

Two clinical studies have shown St. John's wort to be as effective as the prescription drug Tofranil (imipramine), one of the most frequently prescribed tricyclic antidepressants. At the Imerem Institute for Medical Research Management and Biometrics in Nuremberg, Germany, psychiatry professor Michael Philipp, M.D. and colleagues gave 1,050 milligrams of standardized St. John's wort extract, Tofranil, or a placebo daily for eight weeks to 263 patients suffering from moderate depression. The results showed that St. John's wort was superior to the placebo and comparable to the drug in relieving the patients' symptoms as measured by the Hamilton Anxiety Scale, the Clinical Global Impression Scale, and the Zung Self-Rating Depression Scale. The patients who were given St. John's wort had one-third the incidence of side effects as those taking Tofranil; the chief side effect reported was dry mouth. The researchers noted that St. John's wort is a safe treatment for depression and that it improves quality of life for patients.

In another German study, Helmut Woelk, M.D. and colleagues at the University of Giessen gave 500 milligrams of standardized St. John's wort or Tofranil daily for six weeks to 324 patients with mild to moderate depression. Both the herb and the drug decreased the patients' symptoms of depression by half. St. John's wort, however, surpassed Tofranil in reducing symptoms of anxiety. The researchers also noted that almost half of the study participants experienced side effects while taking Tofranil (primarily dry mouth and nausea), whereas only 20 percent of those taking St. John's wort experienced side effects (most commonly dry mouth).

In addition, an overview published in 1996 in the *British Medical Journal* evaluated twenty-three clinical trials involving a total of 1,757 outpatients with mild to moderately severe depressive disorders. The report concluded that St. John's wort extracts were significantly superior to a placebo in relieving depression and as effective as standard antidepressants.

Challenge to St. John's Wort

In 2001, a study published in the *Journal of the American Medical Association* disputed the effectiveness of St. John's wort and ensuing newspaper headlines reported that the herb had been found useless for the treatment of depression. It turned out, however, that this study was very misleading, as it was conducted with a group of patients suffering from severe depression. St. John's wort has never been touted as the most effective treatment for severe depression; rather, it has been recommended for treating mild to moderate cases of depression, for which numerous clinical studies have demonstrated not only that it is as effective as prescription antidepressants but also that its side effects are far fewer and much less severe. (Even this controversial report acknowledged that a few of the patients suffering from severe depression did benefit from taking St. John's wort. It is also important to note that this study was funded and organized by Pfizer, the same pharmaceutical company that makes Zoloft, which is one of the most often prescribed conventional antidepressant drugs.)

How to Use St. John's Wort

St. John's wort is available in many different forms including teas, capsules, tablets, and liquid extracts; it has traditionally been used as a tea and as a tincture (a liquid extract made by crushing and steeping the herb in food-grade alcohol). Teas made from St. John's wort are not recommended for treating depression, because the presumed active ingredient(s) are not adequately extracted in hot water. Tinctures, which are labeled as liquid extracts by manufacturers, effectively extract the active chemicals. Of course, this depends on the initial quality of the plant material and the care of the manufacturer during processing, so the amount of active ingredients can vary greatly in liquid extracts. If you want to try a nonstandardized liquid extract of St. John's wort, the Herb Research Foundation in Boulder, Colorado suggests taking twenty to thirty drops three times a day, diluted in a small amount of juice or warm water, with meals.

All of the research on St. John's wort has been conducted with standardized extracts (either as capsules or tablets), which makes it easier for researchers to maintain consistency in their studies. Although St. John's wort products do not have to be standardized to be effective, buy standardized extracts if you want to be sure that you are obtaining adequate levels of the active compounds. St. John's wort extracts are typically standardized to contain 0.3% hypericin and 5% hyperforin.

Most of the research on St. John's wort has used 900 milligrams daily (usually taken as 300 milligrams three times a day). Some people respond well to lesser amounts of the herb and others need more; you can adjust the dosage as needed. It's safe to take as much as 1,800 milligrams of St. John's wort daily but you should first use the herb for at least two months at the standard daily dose of 900 milligrams. To increase the amount, add an additional 300 milligrams daily for one month and then continue each month to add an additional 300 milligrams to your daily dose as you feel is necessary (stop adding if you reach 1,800 milligrams). Working with a health practitioner who is familiar with St. John's wort can be helpful in determining the dosage that is most appropriate for you.

It's best to take St. John's wort in three equal doses, one with each meal. Taking the herb with a meal helps prevent the possibility of digestive upset and taking it at regular intervals throughout the day keeps a steady supply of the active ingredients available to your body.

What to Expect and How Long to Take St. John's Wort

Many people notice a significant difference within a couple of weeks of using St. John's wort and report improvements in sleep quality, energy levels, and appetite—but don't be discouraged if you don't notice changes right away, as the full effects of St. John's wort can take several weeks to kick in. The most common mistake that people make when taking herbal supplements is giving the herb insufficient time to have a physiological effect on the body. You should expect results but be patient and take the herb for at least six weeks before making a decision about whether or not to continue it.

It's also important to take St. John's wort regularly, not just when you are feeling depressed. The herb has a cumulative positive effect on depression, so interrupting your regular dosage schedule can diminish the benefits. Don't worry, however, if you happen to miss a dose; just try to keep as much as possible to a regular schedule of taking the herb and you can double up on a dose if necessary. If you don't see positive results from St. John's wort within six to eight weeks, it's possible that the supplement you are taking may not contain adequate amounts of the active compounds to be effective. For this reason, it is essential to buy quality herbal products from a reputable company (see the Appendix). Ask a doctor, pharmacist, or qualified herbalist for recommendations.

As your depression lifts and your sleep improves, you may want to consider beginning to taper off of St. John's wort. For most people, staying on the herb for at least one month after depressive symptoms have abated is helpful. Although there are generally no negative side effects associated with discontinuing St. John's wort, it's a good idea to do so gradually, lessening your dosage by 300 milligrams at a time over a period of weeks. Many people take St. John's wort for brief periods, whereas others find that they do best when they use the herb for months or even years. St. John's wort can be taken for as long as is necessary and can be used safely for an indefinite period of time (but see Cautions for St. John's Wort, below).

Cautions for St. John's Wort

The long history of safety of St. John's wort makes it a valuable alternative to prescription antidepressants for many people. Side effects occasionally occur with the herb but they are uncommon and tend to be minor. Most people can use St. John's wort safely. As with any medicinal herb or drug, certain precautions should be observed.

- If you are taking St. John's wort, be sure to tell your doctor, because the herb may affect other medications that you are taking (see the inset "Effect of St. John's Wort on Prescription Drugs" on page 81).

- If you are pregnant, do not take St. John's wort without consulting your doctor.

- Some people report mild stomach upset while using the herb. Taking St. John's wort with food can help prevent digestive upset.

- More rarely, some people experience allergic reactions, fatigue, or restlessness while using St. John's wort. If you notice any of these symptoms, consult your healthcare practitioner for advice before continuing to use the herb.

Effect of St. John's Wort on Prescription Drugs

Research reported by the National Institutes of Health in early 2000 revealed that St. John's wort may reduce the effectiveness of some prescription drugs. St. John's wort appears to speed up activity in a key metabolic pathway that is responsible for the breakdown of various medications; in other words, the herb causes the body to process the drugs more quickly, which then lowers blood levels of the medications and decreases their effectiveness.

As a result, the U.S. FDA asked healthcare professionals to caution patients about the potential risks of combining St. John's wort with other medications. This does not mean that St. John's wort can never be used in combination with any prescription drugs. It simply means that, in order to be safe and to avoid harmful drug interactions, you should always let your doctor know about any herbs and supplements you may be using.

Specifically, St. John's wort has been found to affect indinavir and other protease inhibitors, which are antiviral drugs used to treat HIV infection. The herb also apparently affects cyclosporin, which is used to help prevent organ rejection in transplant patients. In addition, it may affect other immunosuppressant drugs that work through the same pathway; these include birth control pills, cholesterol-lowering medications such as Mevacor (lovastatin), heart-disease medications such as digoxin, some cancer medications, anti-seizure medications, and blood thinners such as Coumadin (warfarin). If you are taking any of these drugs, taking St. John's wort may interfere with their effectiveness and could potentially be dangerous.

- St. John's wort is classified as toxic to livestock because it can cause severe photosensitivity (an adverse reaction to sunlight) in animals grazing on the herb. Although this reaction is uncommon in humans, there have been a few reports of photosensitivity in people taking therapeutic amounts of St. John's wort. Symptoms of photosensitivity include skin rash, unusual susceptibility to sunburn, or pain or burning of the skin when exposed to ultraviolet light. Fair-skinned people are most vulnerable, as are people who have experienced reactions to ultraviolet light when taking other types of medications. Take care to avoid excessive sun exposure, tanning lamps, and other sources of ultraviolet light while taking St. John's wort.

- If you are currently taking antidepressant medications, it is essential that you work with your doctor if you are interested in taking St. John's wort. Do not attempt to abruptly discontinue antidepressants; instead, work with your doctor to gradually wean yourself from prescription medications. Also, be aware that in some cases (especially for people with major chronic depression and those with bipolar disorder), prescription medications are probably necessary.

8

Special Supplements for Specific Sleep-Related Problems: Melatonin and 5-HTP

It seems like a sensible idea to try to improve health and well-being by supplementing the body's supply of nutritional building blocks such as vitamins and minerals; it can be difficult to take this approach, however, with compounds that are produced or utilized by the brain. Fortunately for many people who struggle with sleep problems, it is possible to supplement our innate supply of certain substances that are involved in the brain's regulation of the sleep/ wake cycle. In this chapter, you'll learn more about the hormone melatonin and a compound with the strange-sounding name of 5-hydroxytryptophan.

Melatonin has gotten a lot of press in recent years as a treatment for jet lag, insomnia, and even aging. This fascinating hormone appears to have a number of health benefits and research is continuing to determine exactly how melatonin works and for what conditions it is beneficial. Thus far, a number of studies have verified that melatonin is an effective aid for many sleep disorders. 5-hydroxytryptophan or 5-HTP is a chemical naturally produced by the body that plays an essential role in the regulation of mood and sleep. Taking supplements of 5-HTP can help relieve insomnia and can also help lift the depression that often contributes to sleep disorders.

WHAT IS MELATONIN?

Until fairly recently, the purpose of the pineal gland, a pea-sized structure at the base of the brain, was a mystery to scientists. This gland is now recognized, however, as a key player in regulating certain hormones and setting our biological clocks. Our circadian rhythms are established by the ebb and flow of melatonin, which is secreted by the pineal gland and has a particularly important role in regulating the sleep/wake cycle. In fact, melatonin can be thought of as the body's natural sleep-aid.

The production of this hormone is a complex dance that closely ties us to the rising and setting of the sun. During the day, melatonin levels in the body are so low that it's difficult to detect any; but at dusk, the decreasing light triggers the pineal gland to begin secreting the hormone. In accordance with interrelated circadian rhythms, body temperature starts to drop and alertness wanes as your body prepares for rest. During the night as you sleep, melatonin flows through the bloodstream, with its level peaking at about 2:00 A.M. in healthy young people and at about 3:00 A.M. in elderly people. After peaking, melatonin levels quickly decline, which helps the body prepare to awaken in the morning.

Children have the greatest amounts of melatonin but its production begins a sharp decline at puberty. Thereafter, the amount of melatonin produced by the pineal gland varies widely among individuals; for some, levels of the hormone diminish significantly with age, which may be the reason that many people have difficulty sleeping as they get older. Supplemental melatonin can help improve sleep quality and restore a normal sleep/wake cycle, thereby enhancing overall quality of life. Melatonin supplementation is especially useful for people whose natural sleep pattern has been disrupted by factors such as jet lag, seasonal affective disorder (SAD), shift work, and possibly depression (see Chapters 2 and 3).

Research continues into melatonin and its relationship to many aspects of health. Studies indicate that this important hormone may inhibit the development of atherosclerosis, reduce blood triglyceride levels, and enhance immunity. Animal studies have even suggested that melatonin has the potential to increase lifespan.

How Melatonin Works

Jet lag from time-zone changes is a common cause of circadian rhythm disturbances but anything that interferes with normal sleep patterns results in a comparable physiological trauma. Working the night shift or even simply staying up all night causes symptoms similar to jet lag (see Sleep Problems of Modern Life on page 17) because the body's production of melatonin is affected, upsetting the biological clock. Many other things including emotional stress and aging can influence melatonin production.

A lack of this important hormone negatively affects numerous mental and physiological functions. For example, memory, decision-making, and clarity of thinking are all profoundly affected by a decrease in melatonin. Scientists now know that the melatonin pulse—that is, the rate at which melatonin is secreted—is intimately involved in regulating the neuroendocrine system. Fatigue, insomnia, headache, irritability, constipation, and reduced immunity are also common side effects when the biological clock is thrown off-kilter.

Like most physiological processes, the melatonin pulse varies from individual to individual. You can manipulate the lightness and darkness in your environment to help increase your body's natural production of this critical hormone. Because the amount of melatonin secreted varies according to the amount of light that you are exposed to, your pineal gland will produce more melatonin if you sleep in a completely dark room. To make your bedroom as dark as possible, invest in room-darkening shades or curtains or use a sleep mask that covers your eyes (an excellent solution for traveling, when you might not be able to control the amount of light in the room). Spending time in sunlight every day—preferably in the morning— also helps regulate the production of melatonin.

Many people have found that using supplemental melatonin helps reestablish a healthy circadian rhythm, which facilitates better sleep patterns and sounder sleep. Taking melatonin at night also appears to enhance alertness the following day, as well as lessening mid-afternoon fatigue and the desire to nap.

Scientific Support for Melatonin

Many scientific studies have proven that melatonin is helpful for reestablishing normal sleep patterns, especially when circadian rhythms have been disrupted by schedule irregularities or simply by the natural process of aging.

In a 1998 double-blind experiment reported in *Chronobiology International*, researchers evaluated 320 people divided into four groups who received a daily dose of 5 milligrams of standard melatonin, 5 milligrams of slow-release melatonin, $1/2$ milligram of standard melatonin, or a placebo, for four days following airplane travel. The group given 5 milligrams of standard melatonin took less time to fall asleep, slept better, and was more energetic during the day than the other three groups. Another double-blind study, this time of airplane crews, found that the participants rested better when given 10 milligrams of melatonin as compared to a placebo and that the results with melatonin were as good as with the prescription sedative zoplicone.

A number of researchers have found melatonin to be helpful for improving sleep in the elderly, who frequently experience sleep disturbances; studies have attributed various benefits, including falling asleep more readily and decreased middle-of-the-night awakenings, to melatonin supplementation. Melatonin is also beneficial for children who are troubled by chronic sleep disturbance. In 2001, a double-blind investigation published in the *Journal of Child Neurology* evaluated forty children who had trouble falling asleep at night for at least one year prior to the study. The children were given 5 milligrams of melatonin or a placebo for four weeks and those given melatonin experienced significant improvement, being able to fall asleep more easily. *Note:* The long-term safety of melatonin supplementation has not yet been established (see the inset "Caution for Long-Term Use of Melatonin" on page 88). If you wish to use melatonin for a child's sleep difficulty, always check first with your doctor.

In one interesting study, researchers found that melatonin is even useful for the legions of people who stay up late on weekends and then have trouble going to sleep at a reasonable hour on Sunday night. The researchers found that the optimal time for taking melatonin in such cases of "weekend insomnia" is about five and one-half hours prior to the time you wish to go to sleep on Sunday night.

Melatonin supplements have also been shown to be helpful for people who wish to wean themselves from conventional sleeping medications. In a double-blind study reported in 1999 in the journal *Archives of Internal Medicine,* thirty-four people regularly taking benzodiazepine sedatives were able to stop using the drugs by taking 2 milligrams nightly of melatonin. *Note:* If you are currently taking prescription sedatives and are interested in switching to melatonin, consult your doctor first (see Cautions for Melatonin on page 88).

How to Use Melatonin

Supplemental melatonin is manufactured either naturally or synthetically. Natural melatonin is derived from extracts of animal pineal glands. In this case, natural is not better, because animal tissue can be contaminated with viruses. Synthetic or pharmacy-grade melatonin is molecularly identical to natural melatonin but is made in the laboratory and is free of animal tissue.

Melatonin is available in two forms: standard melatonin, which is sometimes called "quick release"; and "slow release" (also called "controlled release"), which releases small amounts of the hormone over a number of hours. Some research indicates that quick-release melatonin facilitates falling asleep more quickly and that slow-release melatonin aids in staying asleep. The best approach to using melatonin for your sleep problem may be to try one form and then, if it doesn't produce the desired results, to try the alternate form.

The most important consideration in using melatonin is the time that you take it. Melatonin should always be taken at night and preferably before midnight, because that's when the pineal gland naturally secretes the hormone. By correctly scheduling your intake of supplemental melatonin in the evening, you help quickly reset and maintain healthy internal rhythms and can even prevent jet lag and similar circadian rhythm disturbances. If you take melatonin after midnight, you run the risk of further upsetting your body's internal clock and you may find that you've inadvertently created temporary symptoms of jet lag.

For best results, take melatonin approximately thirty minutes to one hour before you wish to go to sleep; remember to take it according to your desired bedtime in whichever time zone you're visiting. If you're traveling for a period of several days or longer or traveling across several time zones, use it for four to five days or until you feel acclimated to the local time. Even if you're only treating a "simple" case of jet lag, take melatonin for four to five days following your flight; for the majority of people, this is sufficient time for the biological clock to reset itself. Most people who take melatonin wake up feeling refreshed the next day—of course, you may still feel some residual fatigue simply from the stress of travel.

Appropriate doses of melatonin vary from person to person because of individual differences in absorption and metabolism of the hormone. Researchers have not determined an optimal dose but in general, most people experience positive results with 1–10 milligrams of melatonin for jet lag or other causes of insomnia. Start by taking 3 milligrams; if you sleep well but are drowsy in the morning, cut the dose in half; if, on the other hand, your sleep doesn't improve, increase your dose by 3 milligrams each night (stopping at the upper limit of 10 milligrams) until you achieve the desired effect.

Caution for Long-Term Use of Melatonin

Further study is needed to determine the effects of supplemental melatonin when it is used over a long period of time. Until more is known, it's important to remember that melatonin is a hormone and that hormones have a powerful influence on the body. Cumulative results of the long-term use of hormones can sometimes take years to become evident. Taking supplemental melatonin may also affect the levels of other hormones in the body. If you're planning to use melatonin for more than a few weeks, it's a good idea to do so under the supervision of your doctor, who can help you monitor its effects.

Cautions for Melatonin

Melatonin is generally regarded as a safe dietary supplement (but see the inset "Caution for Long-Term Use of Melatonin" above). Researchers have administered a wide range of melatonin dosages to study participants, with no negative effects. As noted previously, however, people vary in the amount of melatonin that is optimal for their needs. It's best to start with a low dose and to increase your dose only if necessary. Review the following cautions when taking melatonin.

- Taking too much melatonin can cause sleepiness the next day, headache, depression, or intestinal discomfort.

- Obviously, as melatonin is taken to induce sleep, drowsiness and a decrease in attention can be expected as normal side effects of the hormone. Therefore, you should not drive or operate machinery for several hours after taking melatonin.

- If you are pregnant or nursing or have any chronic illness, check with your doctor before taking melatonin.

- If you are currently taking prescription sedatives and are interested in switching to melatonin, consult your doctor for advice about how to proceed.

WHAT IS 5-HTP?

The supplemental form of 5-hydroxytryptophan (5-HTP) is derived from the seed of an African plant called griffonia (*Griffonia simplicifolia*). In the body, 5-HTP is created as a product of the metabolism of the amino acid tryptophan, when tryptophan is broken down to make the neurotransmitter serotonin. As previously mentioned, neurotransmitters are compounds that facilitate communication between nerve cells and are involved in regulating various bodily functions. Serotonin has an enormous effect on how you feel. It controls mood, eating behavior, and sleep and also regulates the activity of many other neurotransmitters. The role that 5-HTP plays as a precursor to serotonin is the reason that taking supplemental 5-HTP can help with sleep disorders.

With an adequate supply of serotonin in your brain, you feel calm, relaxed, and patient. Other characteristics of sufficient serotonin include the ability to concentrate, feelings of optimism, sleeping well with good dream recall, and not overeating carbohydrates. If you have too little serotonin, you will likely feel depressed, anxious, and irritable, crave sweets and high-carbohydrate foods, suffer from insomnia, and have poor dream recall. The lower your brain level of serotonin, the more severe these physical and emotional symptoms tend to be. However, the problems that occur with serotonin deficiency vary according to our biochemical individuality and not everyone experiences the same constellation of symptoms. Although exhibiting every characteristic of serotonin deficiency is unlikely, you are likely to suffer from more than one if your serotonin level is low.

Because serotonin can only be manufactured by the body, supplements of serotonin don't exist. However, you can increase your serotonin level by providing your body with more of the materials it needs for making this important neurotransmitter, which is where supplemental 5-HTP can help.

How 5-HTP Works

Researchers believe that by stimulating the production of serotonin, supplementing with 5-HTP corrects deficiencies caused by long-term stress. Many antidepressant drugs work similarly by increasing serotonin levels in the brain (see Antidepressants on page 124). Supplemental 5-HTP has primarily been used for depression but it has also been found effective in treating other disorders that often accompany depression: for example, insomnia, anxiety, chronic migraine headaches, fibromyalgia, and some cases of obesity.

The link between 5-HTP and insomnia appears to be straightforward. The body converts tryptophan into 5-HTP, converts 5-HTP into serotonin (which is itself a sleep/wake regulator), and then changes some of the serotonin into the hormone melatonin. As discussed earlier in this chapter, melatonin helps regulate the body's internal clock and is essential for sleep as well.

Scientific Support for 5-HTP

Several small, short-term studies have found 5-HTP to be as effective against depression as standard antidepressant drugs. In one six-week study, researchers gave sixty-three participants either 100 milligrams of 5-HTP three times daily or 50 milligrams of fluvoxamine (a prescription antidepressant) three times daily; 5-HTP was as effective as the drug but had fewer side effects. Additionally, a review of thirty-seven studies reported in 2000 in *The Alternative Medicine Review* indicated that 5-HTP is beneficial for patients with mild to moderate depression. Three studies in that review also showed that 200–600 milligrams of 5-HTP was specifically helpful for improving sleep quality, primarily by increasing REM sleep.

Because of its effects on serotonin levels, 5-HTP is a helpful supplement for people suffering from chronic fatigue and fibromyalgia as well; low levels of serotonin are associated with more severe physical and emotional symptoms in these conditions. Research indicates, for example, that 5-HTP increases levels of pain tolerance in people with fibromyalgia. In a double-blind study of fifty fibromyalgia sufferers, those who took 100 milligrams of 5-HTP three times a day for thirty days reported a significant decrease in pain and number of tender points; an improvement in sleep; and a reduction in morning stiffness, fatigue, and anxiety.

The picture of 5-HTP's effectiveness for anxiety treatment is not as clear. In a double-blind study of forty-five people suffering from anxiety disorders, participants were given either 5-HTP or the anti-anxiety drug clomipramine for eight weeks. Although the researchers found that 5-HTP was effective, clomipramine helped even more to relieve anxiety symptoms. When choosing between drug therapy and supplemental 5-HTP, however, it's important to consider that the side effects of 5-HTP are fewer and less severe (see Chapter 12).

How to Use 5-HTP

Using supplemental 5-HTP sometimes causes mild nausea during the first several weeks of taking it. Starting with a low dose lessens the likelihood of nausea, as does taking 5-HTP along with food. You might also consider using enteric-coated 5-HTP capsules or tablets, which decrease the potential for stomach upset.

For treating depression, begin by taking 50 milligrams of 5-HTP three times daily, with meals or snacks. If you don't see results within two weeks, increase the dosage to 100 milligrams three times per day. For treating insomnia, begin by taking 100 milligrams of 5-HTP at thirty to forty-five minutes before bed. If you don't see results within a few days, then gradually increase the dosage as necessary in 50-milligram increments, up to a total of 300 milligrams per day. For treating fibromyalgia, begin by taking 50 milligrams of 5-HTP three times daily with food. If you don't see results within two weeks, increase the dosage to 100 milligrams three times per day.

Cautions for 5-HTP

Although no significant side effects other than initial mild nausea have commonly been associated with the use of 5-HTP, one report several years ago indicated that some batches of the supplement were contaminated

Tryptophan, 5-HTP, and Peak X Contamination

A toxic compound was found in some batches of tryptophan, an amino-acid supplement that was widely used for a number of years for treating depression and insomnia. In 1989, tryptophan was taken off the market after a contaminated batch was linked to a serious blood disorder called eosinophiliamyalgia syndrome (EMS) in approximately 1,500 people, resulting in thirty-eight deaths. Many experts believe that a chemical called Peak X, introduced by a manufacturing error, was the cause of the disorder.

Because supplemental 5-HTP is manufactured completely differently than supplemental tryptophan, it is unlikely that the same risk of contamination could occur. Although there was apparently one incident of contamination of 5-HTP in 1994, there have been no further occurrences and manufacturers have since taken precautions to ensure that their 5-HTP supplements do not contain Peak X.

with a harmful chemical called Peak X (see the inset "Tryptophan, 5-HTP, and Peak X Contamination" on page 91). Although 5-HTP is considered safe, you should review the following precautions before using it.

- If you are taking prescription antidepressants or other drugs that raise serotonin levels (including anti-migraine drugs in the triptan family), do not use 5-HTP without first consulting your doctor. Supplemental 5-HTP may intensify the effects of drugs that increase serotonin. Too much serotonin can cause "serotonin syndrome," producing symptoms such as agitation, rapid heart rate, high blood pressure, loss of coordination, and confusion.

- If you are taking carbidopa, often prescribed for Parkinson's disease, 5-HTP may cause changes in the skin that are similar to the thickening and hardening that occurs in a disease called scleroderma.

- If you are pregnant or nursing, consult your healthcare practitioner before taking 5-HTP.

9

Simple Behavioral and Cognitive Strategies for a Better Night's Sleep

As you've discovered in Chapters 1 through 4 of this book, sleep problems are caused by a wide variety of factors. Whether a sleep problem is the result of stress, lifestyle issues, or a physical or psychological condition, therapies that focus on behavioral and cognitive changes are almost always helpful. The successful treatment of your insomnia may require identifying and changing the behaviors or even the thought patterns that are interfering with your sleep.

Behavioral and cognitive treatments for insomnia are specifically designed to train people in the art of sleeping well. In this chapter, you'll learn about several such approaches to sleep improvement. Some of the techniques are simple anxiety- and stress-relieving exercises that you can practice at bedtime, while others are comprehensive cognitive-behavioral programs designed to relieve more deeply entrenched sleep disorders.

BEHAVIORAL CHANGES AND INSOMNIA

Researchers have found that behavioral therapies for insomnia are more effective than drugs for all age groups, including the elderly, who typically have the most problems with sleep disturbances. Studies show that at least three-quarters of insomnia patients treated with behavioral and other non-drug therapies report sleep improvement—and this is with an average treatment duration of only one month. Studies have also shown that the majority of people who rely on drugs to induce sleep are able to completely stop or at least reduce their use of sleeping medications after treatment with behavioral methods.

But do these behavioral techniques work over the long term? In a study published in 1999 in the *Journal of the American Medical Association*, drug treatment was compared to cognitive/behavioral therapy for seventy-eight insomnia patients with a mean age of sixty-five. The participants were given eight weeks of treatment with drugs, cognitive/behavioral therapy, or a combination of the two. The researchers found that all three groups experienced short-term sleep improvement but then at two-year follow-up, they found that those patients who had received cognitive/behavioral therapy with or without drug treatment were best able to maintain their improvements. Clearly, preventing or overcoming a sleep disorder can depend, in a number of cases, on an individual's ability to relax and to learn healthy sleep patterns.

Sleep Hygiene

The simplest strategy of all for healthy sleep is referred to as sleep hygiene, which encompasses the most basic activities and behaviors that promote good sleep. In fact, practicing good sleep hygiene is beneficial for anyone interested in ensuring the most restful sleep possible. Applying the following principles of sleep hygiene should be the first approach when dealing with any type of sleep problem.

- Establish a regular time for going to bed and another for getting up in the morning and adhere to those times as much as possible, even on weekends and during vacations. Although it's tempting to try to make up for lost sleep by sleeping in whenever you have the opportunity, it's more important to train your body to wake at a consistent time so that you will be ready to go to sleep at your designated bedtime.

- Use your bed only for sleep and sexual relations. Avoid being in bed during activities such as watching television, working, studying, eating, or making phone calls. These pursuits stimulate alertness instead of allowing the body and mind to relax and prepare for sleep.

- Make sure that your bedroom is a comfortable temperature (slightly on the cool side usually works best: see Your Surroundings and Your Sleep on page 16) and well-ventilated. In addition, make sure that your bedroom is completely dark, which stimulates the production of melatonin and deep, restorative sleep.

- Avoid taking naps during the day. Napping may seem like a good idea if you're sleep deprived but napping actually contributes to the problem of nighttime insomnia. Remember that the goals of sleep hygiene are to train your body to sleep at night and to establish and maintain a regular sleep pattern.

- Exercise daily, at least thirty minutes a day. Regular exercise is an excellent way to alleviate stress, anxiety, and depression. Studies have found that exercise is as beneficial as prescription drugs for promoting sleep (see Chapter 10). But avoid exercising—especially vigorous exercise—within three hours of bedtime or you may find that you are too energized to sleep.

- Cultivate the habit of doing something relaxing in the hour before bedtime. Read a novel, listen to soothing music, meditate, or practice calming yoga poses (see Chapters 10 and 11).

- At an hour or two before bedtime, soak in a hot bath. This leads to a change in your core body temperature and facilitates relaxation. But don't soak in a hot bath immediately prior to bedtime, because the extreme heat can stimulate alertness that you don't want to experience while you're trying to get to sleep. A warm Epsom salts bath just before bed, however, can be deeply relaxing (see Hydrotherapy on page 115).

- Go to bed at your prescribed bedtime but then ignore the clock. Turn the clock face to the wall so that you won't know what time it is. If you're having trouble going to sleep, fretting over the time will exacerbate the problem.

- Make sure to eat dinner at least three hours before bedtime to give your body time to digest the meal before you try to sleep. This precaution also helps prevent gastroesophageal reflux (see Chapter 3), which can cause nighttime heartburn. A light snack before bed, however, can promote sleep onset and prevent nocturnal dips in blood sugar that trigger middle-of-the-night awakenings (see Dietary Suggestions for Better Sleep on page 44). Avoid sugary bedtime snacks, though, as these can wreak havoc with blood sugar levels.

- Avoid drinking too much liquid in the hour before bedtime to prevent having to get up during the night to urinate.

- Stay away from caffeine in all of its forms: coffee, tea, chocolate, soft drinks, and certain over-the-counter medications (check your prescription medications for caffeine, too). Caffeine not only causes difficulties in going to sleep but can also cause awakening in the night. The stimulating effects of caffeine can last up to twenty-four hours, so it's a good idea to eliminate it from your life completely if you have chronic trouble sleeping (see Caffeine and Insomnia on page 56).

- Don't overdo alcohol. Although alcohol has an initial sedative effect that lasts for several hours, it can then cause restless sleep and frequent awakening during the night (see Subtle Sleep Disruptors on page 55). Limit your daily alcohol intake to one drink or a glass of wine or beer with dinner.

- If you smoke, quit. Along with all of the other health detriments of smoking, nicotine is a stimulant that interferes with sleep.

- Spend time in sunlight every day—approximately one-half hour—to help regulate your body's production of the hormones (like melatonin: see Chapters 1 and 8) that support sleep. It's best to get your sun exposure early in the day, which is the time that is most effective for regulating your body's internal clock and is also the safest time for your skin to be in the sun.

- If you're having trouble sleeping fifteen or twenty minutes after going to bed, get up, go into another room, and read, listen to soothing music, or engage in some other quiet activity in dim lighting until you begin to feel sleepy. Don't watch television; it's too stimulating and the bright light will trigger wakefulness. If for some reason you are physically unable to get out of bed, keep a boring book by the side of your bed and read by a low-intensity light.

- If you have chronic problems sleeping, you might want to consider sleeping alone, at least on nights that you're suffering from insomnia. Sleeping alone is generally more restful than sleeping with a partner.

Stimulus Control Therapy

Many times, people who have trouble sleeping develop an adverse reaction to sleep even though they feel tired. Because of previous negative experiences, they associate getting into bed with having problems sleeping and therefore become anxious instead of relaxed at bedtime. Lying awake and worrying about not being able to sleep further entrenches this form of insomnia.

Many sleep therapists recommend stimulus control therapy, which focuses on breaking the negative thought patterns associated with learned insomnia. The basic principles of stimulus control therapy are to learn to associate the bedroom with sleep and to eliminate the activities or situations that trigger wakefulness. The protocol (see below) includes some of the same recommendations for good sleep hygiene that were given previously in this chapter. As an adjunct to the stimulus control approach, techniques such as progressive muscle relaxation (see Chapter 10) or meditation (see Chapter 11) can be very helpful for reducing the anxiety or stress that perpetuates learned insomnia.

- To help reestablish a regular, healthy sleep/wake cycle, go to bed only in the evening and only when you are sleepy.

- If you suffer from any type of insomnia, it's essential to use your bedroom for sleep and sex only. Don't watch television, read, eat, or work in the bedroom, because all of these stimulating activities encourage wakefulness.

- If you haven't fallen asleep within fifteen to twenty minutes after going to bed, get up, go into a room with dim lighting, and do something relaxing. The best activities for this time are those that promote calmness and aren't too engaging; try reading something boring, listening to soothing music, or unwinding with a relaxation tape. As soon as you become sleepy, return to your bedroom and go back to bed.

- If you awaken during the night and are unable to get back to sleep within fifteen to twenty minutes, repeat the same procedure as above. In the early stages of stimulus control therapy, you might need to get up several times or more during the night. To be successful, you must be persistent.

- It's essential to maintain a regular time of rising in the morning, no matter how little sleep you may have had during the night. It's probably best to set an alarm to help you wake up. This morning waketime regularity will help reset your biological clock and train your body to sleep at night.

- For the same reason, avoid napping during the day. Naps, especially afternoon and evening naps, interfere with nighttime sleep because the ease of sleep onset is directly related to how much time has elapsed since the last sleep period.

Sleep Restriction Therapy

In some tough cases of insomnia, especially when sleep hygiene, stimulus control therapy, and relaxation techniques have not offered sufficient relief, sleep restriction therapy can be useful. Like stimulus control therapy, sleep restriction therapy is based on the idea that time spent in bed worrying about sleep causes increased anxiety and aggravation that further interfere with the ability to sleep. The strategy behind this systematic approach, however, is to transform that frustrating, fragmented time into productive, peaceful sleep by limiting the time spent in bed to a few hours per night, creating mild sleep deprivation, which generally makes it easier to fall asleep. As sleep onset and continuity improve, the length of time spent in bed is then gradually lengthened until a full night of restful sleep is obtained. Although sleep restriction may seem at first to be the opposite of what is needed by someone with insomnia, it can actually be very helpful for reestablishing a healthy sleeping pattern.

The first step in sleep restriction therapy is to calculate your sleep efficiency number. To do this, keep a sleep diary for two weeks, recording for every night the hours that you spend in bed and the actual hours that you spend sleeping. Determine your average hours spent sleeping per night and your average hours spent in bed per night; then, divide your average nightly sleeping hours by your average nightly hours in bed. The result is your sleep efficiency number, which is given as a percentage. For example, if you average eight hours in bed but are asleep for an average of only six of those hours, divide six by eight, which equals .75, which is a sleep efficiency value of 75 percent. The goal of sleep restriction therapy is to achieve a sleep efficiency of 85 to 90 percent—that is, being awake for only 10 to 15 percent of your total time in bed.

Initially, you must gradually reduce the amount of time you spend in bed. The first week, begin by going to bed fifteen minutes later than your usual bedtime. Continue keeping your sleep diary throughout this treatment so that you can accurately calculate your weekly sleep efficiency. If you still have not reached 85 percent sleep efficiency by the second week, delay your nightly bedtime by an additional fifteen minutes. During this process, it is critical that you consistently rise at the same time each morning.

Continue reducing your time in bed at one-week increments of fifteen minutes, even if you feel tired, until your calculated weekly sleep efficiency becomes 90 percent (but don't decrease your time in bed to less than five

Behavioral Steps Toward Better Sleep

- Go to bed only when you are sleepy.
- Maintain a regular schedule of sleeping and awakening.
- Use your bedroom only for sleep and sex.
- Avoid daytime naps.
- Exercise regularly but avoid vigorous exercise within three hours of bedtime.
- Thirty minutes before bedtime, engage in a relaxing ritual such as reading, listening to music, or taking a warm bath.
- Sleep in a cool, well-ventilated bedroom.
- Avoid large meals within three hours of bedtime.
- Avoid drinking large amounts of fluids one hour before bedtime.
- Avoid caffeine in all forms.
- Avoid nicotine.
- Avoid excessive amounts of alcohol.

hours per night, even if you haven't reached 90 percent efficiency yet). Once you reach the target of 90 percent, you then gradually increase your nightly time in bed by adding fifteen-minute increments each week until your sleep efficiency level begins to drop below 90 percent again. At this point, you will have identified your optimal hours of sleep per night; this should be the amount of sleep that allows you to feel refreshed in the morning.

You can use principles of stimulus control therapy to enhance the process of sleep restriction therapy. For example, if you go to bed and have not fallen asleep within fifteen minutes, get up and do something relaxing. When you again feel sleepy, go back to bed.

COGNITIVE THERAPY AND SLEEP PROBLEMS

Cognitive therapy, which involves identifying the thinking patterns that create emotional stress and anxiety, is often used successfully in treating depression. Learning new ways of thinking to replace negative attitudes with realistic, rational thoughts forms the core of the cognitive approach. Cognitive therapy can also be useful for people who need help changing the thoughts, beliefs, and attitudes that are interfering with healthy sleep patterns. For insomnia, cognitive therapy is usually used in conjunction with behavioral therapies such as stimulus control, relaxation training, and sleep restriction.

Many people have ideas about sleep, based on what they have been taught or what they perceive as "normal," that are unrealistic. For example, most people believe that eight hours of sleep each night is normal and necessary for everyone. The reality is that people vary in the amount of sleep that they need and that quality of sleep is as important as amount. But if you strongly believe that you need eight hours of sleep each night (even though you awaken naturally after seven hours), you might spend an hour in bed fretting about not being able to sleep. If you simply recognize that you are a person who can sleep less than eight hours and still feel well rested, this recognition may be sufficient to relieve the anxiety that you associate with sleeping.

Once an insomnia sufferer becomes aware of the negative thought patterns that contribute to sleep problems, cognitive therapy also includes changing those patterns. For instance, you might have thoughts such as, "I'll never be able to fall asleep tonight" or "I'm always going to have problems sleeping." Learning to counter negative thoughts with positive, realistic statements helps relieve the anxiety that accompanies negative thinking and prevents the creation of a self-fulfilling prophecy of insomnia. Examples of challenges to such negative statements would be, "I can listen to my favorite soothing music, which will help me relax and enable me to sleep" and "I'm learning positive ways of caring for myself so that my body can naturally establish a healthy sleeping pattern."

If worry in general is a contributing factor to your insomnia, you might find it beneficial to set aside a specific time, perhaps in the early evening, to review your day and make plans for the following day. You might also consider keeping a journal, as suggested below. By taking time on a regular basis to "check in" with yourself, you can prevent worrisome thoughts from surfacing later at bedtime and creating anxiety.

Journal Writing for Stress Relief

Journal writing can be a useful technique for helping you to sleep better, especially if anxiety or depression plays a prominent role in your sleep problem. Unexpressed feelings are almost always at the root of emotional pain. Journal writing is a simple yet powerful tool for dissolving emotional blocks and cultivating self-understanding. Journaling can also help you map out a plan for making changes that will result in a more satisfying life and reduce feelings of stress.

By taking time regularly to clear your mind of nagging thoughts and worries, you are likely to sleep more peacefully. Studies have even shown that people who engage in journal writing on a regular basis enhance the functioning of their immune systems and are less prone to illness. Although you don't have to adhere to a schedule to benefit from journal writing, it does help to set aside a consistent time for it. You may find that you enjoy writing in the early morning hours, when your mind is fresh and you can still access insights and images from your dreams; or, you may find that you like to write just before sleeping as a way of processing the day's events. Whatever time you choose, allow yourself at least fifteen minutes to write in your journal.

When you are writing, don't worry about grammar or punctuation. You'll more readily access your feelings if you bypass your intellect. Simply allow the free flow of thoughts and images that arise in your mind to be transferred directly to the paper by your hand. It may take a few journal-writing sessions to feel comfortable writing in this way but you'll soon discover the unique insights into the inner workings of your mind that appear when you allow your thoughts to flow freely onto the paper. As you continue in your process of journal writing, you will strengthen your connection to your inner wisdom, which will help alleviate stress and enhance your overall well-being.

10

Exercise and Relaxation Techniques to Benefit Both Sides of the Sleep/Wake Cycle

E xercise and relaxation therapies, often in conjunction with each other, are useful for easing the muscle tension, physiological and emotional stress, and anxiety that can interfere with sleep. When used prior to bedtime, relaxation exercises help ease physical tension and calm the mind, preparing the body for rest.

In this chapter, you'll learn about mindful exercise, progressive muscle relaxation, breath expansion, and several deceptively simple yoga stretches. The suggestions in this chapter are helpful additions to any program for better sleep in general; several are especially useful for people with particular sleep disorders. Experiment to find the methods that work best for you in promoting better nighttime sleep or counteracting daytime sleepiness. Although most exercise and relaxation techniques take a bit of practice and the commitment to use them regularly in order to be effective, the benefits can be significant.

MINDFUL EXERCISE FOR STRESS RELIEF

One of the quickest ways to relieve tension and anxiety is through exercise, which increases your resistance to stress and helps you adapt to stressors more quickly. Exercise triggers the release of endorphins, the body's natural anxiety-relieving chemicals that enhance mood and feelings of overall well-being. Moderate exercise also metabolizes stress hormones like adrenaline, helping to immediately reduce the physical and emotional impact of stress. Cultivating exercise as a daily habit provides a long-term solution for stress management by preventing physical and mental tension from accumulating.

You can increase the stress-relieving benefits of regular exercise by learning to exercise in a mindful way. Although exercise alone reduces anxiety and strengthens the body against stress-related ills such as high blood pressure and heart disease, combining exercise with aspects of meditation increases the psychological benefits that accompany physical activity. Oftentimes, people who are highly stressed find that they take their problems with them wherever they go, including while they are exercising. Learning to use the power of your mind in a positive way during exercise enables you to attain a state of calmness more quickly. When you exercise mindfully, you also have an opportunity to view the challenges you are encountering in a more positive light.

To practice mindful exercise, it's best to choose a low-intensity aerobic exercise that allows you to move rhythmically and does not require concentration. Walking is ideal but cycling on a stationary bike or swimming laps also works well. Choose a soothing word or a phrase such as a simple prayer or a line from a poem. Some examples are "all is well," "I am safe," "relax," or "peace." As you walk, recite your chosen word or phrase silently in your mind, over and over, in rhythm with your steps. This mental repetition helps quiet the mind and allows you to pay attention to your body's movement and your breathing. When your mind wanders, gently bring your attention back to your steps and continue to repeat your mindful word or phrase. The more you practice, the easier mindful exercise will be, until it becomes natural to leave your worries behind.

Progressive Muscle Relaxation for Insomnia

One of the exercises most commonly prescribed for insomnia is progressive muscle relaxation. This deeply relaxing exercise helps you release tension through a systematic process of contracting and releasing your muscles. The following script describes the practice of progressive muscle relaxation step by step (you might find it easiest to record these instructions on tape and then play the tape when you go to bed at night).

• Lie down in a comfortable position and close your eyes. Take a deep, relaxing breath, expanding your abdomen as you inhale. Exhale completely, allowing your abdomen to sink naturally toward your spine. Take a couple of easy breaths in this way and focus on the rhythm of your breath as it enters and leaves your body. As you exhale, imagine that you are exhaling worries and tension with your breath.

• Consciously focus your attention on your feet. Gently curl your toes as you inhale, hold your inhalation for a moment, and with your next exhalation, relax your feet and toes.

- Move your attention to your lower legs, becoming aware of any tension in your calves. Inhale, flex your feet and gently tense your calves, hold your inhalation for a moment, and as you exhale, relax your calves and feel the tension flowing out of your lower legs and down through your feet.

- Bring your attention to your upper legs and notice any tension that you are holding in your thighs. Inhale while gently tensing your thigh muscles, hold your inhalation for a moment, and then as you exhale, relax your thighs.

- Take another deep, easy breath and feel the tension flowing out of your thighs, down your calves, and out of your feet as you exhale.

- Become aware of your hips and buttocks resting against the surface on which you are lying. Notice any tension that you are holding in your hips and as you inhale, gently tense your buttocks. Hold the tension for a moment and as you exhale, relax your buttocks and hips.

- Focus your attention on your lower back and become aware of tension that you are holding there. Inhale deeply as you gently arch your lower back, hold the inhalation for a moment, and then relax as you release the tension from your lower back.

- Take another deep, relaxing breath and let any remaining tension in your lower back, hips, buttocks, thighs, and calves flow down your legs and out of your feet with your exhalation. Notice and enjoy the feeling of deep relaxation that comes with the release of tension.

- Move your attention to your shoulders and become aware of tension that you are holding there. Inhale and gently tense your shoulder muscles by raising your shoulders toward your ears. Hold the tension for a moment and then release it as you exhale.

- Focus your attention on your upper arms and gently contract the muscles of your upper arms as you inhale. Hold the contraction and then relax and let go of the tension with your exhalation.

- Notice any tension in your lower arms and hands, inhale, and gently curl your hands into fists and tighten the muscles in your forearms. Hold the contraction for a moment and then release it as you exhale.

- Expand your attention to include your shoulders, upper arms, lower arms, and hands, being aware of any remaining tension. Take a deep, relaxing breath and as you exhale, let go of any lingering tension, allowing it to flow down your arms and out of your hands.

- Bring your attention to your upper back, neck, and head and notice the surface upon which your head and upper back are resting. Become aware of any tension that you are holding in your head, neck, and upper back. Contract these muscles as you inhale and hold the contraction for a moment. With a deep exhalation, let the tension flow out of your upper back, neck, and head. Take another deep, relaxing breath and let go of any residual tension.

- Notice any tightness in your forehead and around your eyes and gently tense these muscles as you inhale. Hold the tension for a moment and then release it as you exhale.

- Let your attention move to your mouth and jaw and as you inhale, simply notice any tension there without clenching your jaw. As you exhale, allow your jaw to drop slightly and relax your mouth and jaw completely.

- Take another deep inhalation and hold it for a moment. As you exhale, release any remaining tension in your scalp, face, head, and neck and allow it to flow down through your shoulders, through your arms, and out of your hands and fingers.

- Move your attention to your chest and notice the subtle movement of your chest as you inhale. Take a deep inhalation, expand your chest by gently arching your upper back, and hold the inhalation for a moment. Exhale and let tension flow out of your chest, down your arms, and out through your fingertips.

- Let your attention move to your abdomen and notice how your abdomen expands as you inhale. Inhale deeply, expanding your abdomen fully, and hold the inhalation for a moment. Exhale and let go of any tightness in your abdominal area.

- Inhale a deep, easy breath and imagine your breath filling your entire body with healing relaxation. As you exhale, visualize any remaining tension flowing out of your body. Continue breathing in a relaxed and easy manner for a few minutes, enjoying the deep sense of peace and relaxation that comes from letting go of tension.

Exercise Tips for Specific Sleep Problems

All forms of regular aerobic exercise (including bicycling, dancing, and swimming, for example) are effective for helping to overcome insomnia. Because exercise stimulates production of neurotransmitters that influence mood, sleep patterns, and even pain relief, engaging in regular physical activity can be helpful for alleviating symptoms associated with SAD, chronic fatigue syndrome, fibromyalgia, and menopause; certain exercise suggestions are especially useful against restless legs syndrome and nocturnal leg cramps (see below). In addition, exercising as part of a healthful weight-loss program can improve or even resolve many cases of sleep apnea that are related to excess weight (see Sleep Apnea on page 26).

- **Restless legs syndrome.** Regular moderate exercise—for example, at least thirty minutes of walking or other moderate activity, on most days of the week—is one of the most helpful things you can do to ease restless legs. Avoid long periods of sitting or inactivity and also avoid overly strenuous exercise, which can worsen the symptoms.

- **Nocturnal leg cramps.** If your sleep is disturbed by nocturnal leg cramps, get out of bed and try this calf stretch. Position yourself facing a wall from a couple of feet away, step forward with one foot, and lean toward the wall, placing your forearms and hands firmly against it. Both feet should be pointing toward the wall. Keeping your back leg straight, bend your forward knee and lean further into the wall until you feel a comfortable stretch along the back of the straight leg. Hold the stretch for fifteen to thirty seconds. Switch legs and repeat the calf stretch several times on each side. To prevent muscle cramps, perform this stretch every night before bed.

- **Seasonal affective disorder.** Studies have shown that one of the most powerful tools for overcoming depression is regular aerobic exercise. It generally takes approximately forty-five minutes of moderate aerobic activity to significantly influence mood. If you suffer from SAD, exercising outdoors during daylight hours can be especially helpful for combating depression.

- **Chronic fatigue syndrome and fibromyalgia.** If you suffer from either of these conditions, exercising is probably the last thing you feel like doing but it is essential for regaining your strength and vitality. Walking, biking, and swimming are ideal activities. Start with a reasonable goal (perhaps 10 minutes each day) and then gradually increase your exercise time as your energy level improves. It's important to exercise consistently and moderately—and not to overdo it.

- **Menopause.** Regular exercise is not only beneficial in keeping bones strong but also in relieving the anxiety and mood swings that often accompany menopause. In addition, by helping to regulate hormone levels, exercise helps alleviate hot flashes and insomnia. During the menopausal years, it is optimal to engage in at least thirty minutes of moderate aerobic activity at least five days a week.

BREATHING EXERCISES FOR CALMNESS AND VITALITY

Your breath is one of the most powerful tools you have for relaxing, building vitality, and improving your health. Your breath connects your mind and body; when you purposely focus your attention on breathing more fully and in a more relaxed fashion, you immediately and positively influence your physical and emotional well-being.

Although we think of breathing (if we think of it at all) as an unconscious activity, it often takes conscious practice to transform old breathing habits that contribute to fatigue and tension into new, healthier ways of breathing. Set aside five or ten minutes every day to practice one or more of the following breathing exercises. When you become familiar with the techniques, you can use them anywhere, at any time. Try the deep belly breathing exercise for relaxation and as a natural sleep-aid; or, for an immediate surge of energy, use the energizing breath exercise to quickly increase the level of oxygen in your bloodstream. If you've never before practiced conscious deep breathing, you might initially find that you feel a bit lightheaded. Go slowly with these exercises and work at a pace that feels comfortable to you.

Belly Breathing

Belly breathing, also called diaphragmatic or abdominal breathing, teaches you to breathe correctly. Your abdomen should expand when you inhale and contract when you exhale—but this is actually the opposite of the way that most adults breathe. One of the most common causes of incorrect breathing patterns is chronic stress, which causes shallow upper-chest breathing. To restore a healthful breathing pattern in both wakefulness and sleep, practice the following exercise. You can also perform belly breathing in bed to help prepare your body for rest.

- Lie on your back with your knees bent and your feet flat on the floor about hip-width apart, a comfortable distance from your buttocks. Place your hands on your abdomen to help you feel the expansion and contraction of your abdomen as you breathe.

- Inhale slowly and deeply, allowing your breath to fill and expand your abdomen. As you inhale, gently arch your lower back, which helps expand your abdomen and relax your internal organs.

- Exhale, gently pulling your abdominal muscles in toward your spine, at the same time gently flattening the small of your back against the floor.

- Continue breathing in this way for several minutes and then relax.

Alternate-Nostril Breathing

Alternate-nostril breathing is immensely calming. This exercise helps relax the body and clear the mind of worries. It is helpful to practice alternate-nostril breathing just before bed to facilitate sleep onset if preoccupying thoughts are contributing to sleep problems.

- Sit in a comfortable position with your spine straight and your shoulders relaxed.

- Gently press your right nostril closed with your right thumb and inhale slowly and deeply through your left nostril. Gently press your left nostril closed with the ring finger of your right hand.

- Retain the breath for a few seconds and then release your thumb, exhaling slowly and completely through the right nostril. Immediately inhale through the right nostril with a slow and steady breath.

- Close your right nostril with your right thumb and retain the breath for a few seconds. Release your ring finger and exhale slowly and steadily through your left nostril. Repeat at least ten times, keeping your breath even and controlled.

Relaxing Breath

This easy exercise slows down your breathing and helps you feel calm and relaxed. It's an excellent stress reliever that can be practiced at any time.

- Sit in a comfortable position with your back straight and bring your attention to your breathing.

- Relax and inhale through your nose to a count of five, counting at a pace that is comfortable for you.

- Hold your breath for a count of five.

- Open your mouth slightly and exhale to a count of ten, keeping your exhalation smooth and controlled.

- Repeat the exercise for a total of five complete cycles.

Energizing Breath

This breathing exercise alleviates fatigue and is helpful for providing a boost of energy in the morning or late afternoon.

- Sit with your spine comfortably erect, your feet flat on the floor, and your shoulders relaxed.

- Inhale a series of rapid, short breaths through your nostrils without exhaling, until your lungs are completely filled with air.

- Exhale forcefully through your mouth, making the sound "ha" as you exhale completely.

- Repeat several times and then resume normal breathing.

YOGA FOR DEEP RELAXATION

Yoga is a wonderful form of movement for promoting relaxation. It calms and brings balance to the mind and the body and facilitates emotional and physical harmony through paying attention to the breath. The following are a few simple poses to get you started; for the greatest benefit, find a yoga class with a qualified teacher who can help you learn to perform the movements and postures correctly. To enhance sleep, it's most helpful to practice yoga in the late afternoon or early evening, which helps relieve physical and emotional stresses that have accumulated during the day.

Chest Expander

This yoga exercise loosens tight back and chest muscles and expands your breathing capacity.

- Stand with your spine comfortably straight and your feet about hip-width apart.

- Interlock your fingers behind your back and rest your hands on your buttocks.

- Inhale and raise your arms behind you as high as you comfortably can, keeping your fingers interlocked and your shoulders relaxed.

- Exhale and lower your arms, again resting your hands on your buttocks. Repeat several times.

Child Pose

This calming pose is relaxing for the entire body.

- Kneel on the floor, sitting on your heels with the tops of your feet against the floor. If this feels uncomfortable, wedge a pillow on top of your calves and beneath your thighs, supporting your buttocks with the pillow.

- Bend forward from your hips to place your chest on your knees and your forehead on the floor or on a pillow.

- Stretch your arms out in front of you, palms down, resting on the floor. Alternately, you can place your arms beside your hips with your palms facing up.

- Rest in this position and breathe normally for one minute or as long as you desire.

The Sponge

This deeply restorative and rejuvenating yoga pose is especially relaxing to practice just before bed.

- Lie flat on your back with your legs a comfortable distance apart. Place your arms next to your body with your palms facing up.

- Close your eyes and scan your body for any areas of tension. Consciously relax those areas.

- Use your breath to help you relax. With each inhalation, imagine that you are breathing in relaxation. With each exhalation, imagine that you are breathing out tension.

- Remain in this pose for at least ten minutes.

11

Meditative and Sensory Techniques to Help You Sleep or Wake You Up

Many modern-day therapeutic approaches, including mind-body treatments, are actually connected to healing traditions that have a long history of use in ancient civilizations. In today's fast-paced world, these practices have a renewed relevance for relieving stress and restoring balance to both body and mind. In this chapter, you will learn how meditation, visualization, hydrotherapy, and aromatherapy techniques can be utilized to promote sleep and also to energize you during the day.

MEDITATION

Meditation has been practiced for centuries in many cultural traditions as a way of bringing the body, mind, and spirit into harmonious balance. Basically, meditation involves quieting the mind through gently focused attention. A meditation technique can help you become aware of habitual patterns of thinking and enable you to make better choices about how you are living. Many people find that meditation is an excellent way of relieving stress, because when the mind is calm, the body naturally follows. Obviously, calming the body and mind facilitates restful sleep. The regular practice of meditation also helps you conserve and thereby enhance your energy by helping you approach life in a more relaxed way.

For all forms of meditation, a few basic guidelines will make your experience more beneficial. First, choose a time when your stomach is empty or that's at least one hour after a meal. Many people find early morning or just before bed to be a convenient and beneficial time for meditation. Plan to meditate for fifteen to thirty minutes at a time and establish a regular time and place for your practice. You will enjoy the greatest benefits from meditation when you make it a regular part of your daily life.

Find a quiet place where you will not be disturbed. If you are sitting on a chair, place your feet flat on the floor and sit upright, away from the back of the chair. You can place a firm pillow behind your lower back for support if you wish. If you are sitting on the floor, sit on the edge of a firm cushion to keep your spine erect and cross your legs in a comfortable position. Rest your hands on your thighs or in your lap. Gently close your eyes to help focus your attention inward. Begin each meditation practice with a couple of deep cleansing breaths to release tension from your body.

Meditation on the Breath

Centering your attention on your breath triggers relaxation, calming both body and mind.

- Find a quiet place where you will not be disturbed and sit in a comfortable position. Close your eyes and begin by taking three deep, easy breaths to relax your body, exhaling slowly and completely through your slightly open mouth. Then relax into your normal breathing pattern, inhaling and exhaling through your nose.

- Focus your attention in a gentle way on your breathing. Simply observe your breathing, without trying to change it in any way. As a point of focus, it can be helpful to center your attention on the rising and falling of your abdomen or on your breath as it enters and exits through your nostrils. When your attention wanders, gently bring your focus back to your breath. With practice, your breathing will fall into an easy, natural rhythm. Continue in this way for fifteen to thirty minutes.

- When you are finished with your meditation, expand your attention to include your surroundings and then gently open your eyes.

Mantra Meditation

A mantra is a word or phrase that you silently recite to give your mind a peaceful focus. Choose a word or phrase that has meaning for you; it can be as simple as "peace" or "I am calm." Once you have chosen a mantra and feel satisfied with it, stick with it. It will become associated with the feelings of peace and well-being that you experience during meditation and you will be able to elicit a deep sense of calm at any time by recalling your mantra.

- Sit in a comfortable position, close your eyes, and take three slow, deep breaths, making your exhalation twice as long as your inhalation.

- Focus your attention on your mantra and recite the word or phrase over and over in your mind. Breathe normally and synchronize your mantra with your breathing by repeating it on each exhalation. When your mind wanders, gently bring your attention back to your mantra. Continue your mantra meditation for fifteen to thirty minutes.

- At the end of your meditation, sit quietly for a couple of minutes, expand your attention to include your surroundings, and then gently open your eyes.

VISUALIZATION

Visualization channels the power of your imagination to evoke healthful responses in your mind and body. When you create a mental image of what you would like to manifest, your body and mind respond to the picture as though it were a real experience. When practiced on a regular basis, visualization can improve your health and help you replace negative thought habits with positive, life-affirming ones. You can use the healing visualization technique described below to improve your overall well-being or to focus on a specific health concern (such as a sleep problem). This practice also elicits a state of deep relaxation, which facilitates restful and restorative sleep.

Healing Visualization

The following visualization exercise begins with a deep relaxation that prepares your mind and body to receive the healing images that you create. (You might find it helpful to tape these instructions or have someone read them to you, so that you can fully immerse yourself in the experience without needing to open your eyes to read.)

- Lie in a comfortable position with your eyes closed. Take a deep, easy breath and begin to relax your body and your mind. Focus your attention on your breath, noticing the rising and falling of your abdomen as your breath enters and leaves your body. Without effort, scan your body for tension. Breathe into any tightness that you find and release it with your exhalation. Take three deep, easy breaths, allowing your body and mind to become more deeply relaxed with each exhalation.

- Now imagine in your mind's eye a blank screen. Inhale and visualize the number five on the screen. See the number five clearly in your mind. As you exhale, visualize the number five slowly fading. Take a deep, relaxing inhalation and see the number four appear on the screen in your mind. Exhale and allow the number four to gradually fade. As you inhale again, see the number three appear on the screen. Notice how relaxed you are feeling as you exhale and watch the number three slowly fade. Inhale and visualize the number two on the screen. Exhale, watching the number two fade, and allow yourself to become even more deeply relaxed. Inhale and see the number one appear on the screen. As you exhale completely, watch the number one fade, leaving the screen blank.

- Patiently watch the screen in your mind's eye as an image begins to appear. See yourself on the screen, lying comfortably in a beautiful meadow. It is a warm, sunny day and you are completely safe and protected. Feel the warmth of the sunlight on your body and the gentle breeze caressing your skin. See the rich green of the velvety grass, the deep azure blue of the sky, and the white puffy clouds drifting above you. Smell the sweet freshness of the meadow grasses and flowers and hear the pleasing sounds of the rustle of leaves in the warm breeze, the faint chirping of birds in the trees, and the melodious sound of a gentle nearby stream. Allow yourself to sink even more deeply into this peaceful place, knowing that you are safe and protected. You are warm, comfortable, and completely safe.

- Feel the warmth of the sun and as you inhale, imagine that your body is filled with the golden healing light of the sun's rays. Imagine every cell and organ of your body being bathed, purified, and healed by this warm, soothing light. Notice any place where the energy seems to get stuck and breathe into that place, using your breath and the purifying light to gently dissolve the blockage. Allow the healing energy of the golden light to flow freely throughout your body. Take a few minutes to scan your entire body while you inhale healing, soothing, golden light and exhale tension. Visualize your organs working in perfect harmony and see yourself in vibrant health. Acknowledge the deep relaxation and health that you are experiencing and know that you can access this state of well-being at any time. Relax in this place of balance for a few minutes, enjoying the feeling of being in perfect health.

• When you are ready, take a deep breath and begin to slowly bring your attention back to the present moment. Become aware of your surroundings, stretch your arms and legs, and gently open your eyes while maintaining a feeling of deep calmness and well-being.

HYDROTHERAPY

Hydrotherapy, which means water therapy, is one of the oldest natural healing treatments and has been practiced for centuries by people around the world for relaxation and health improvement. The following simple hydrotherapy techniques can be used to stimulate blood and lymph circulation, ease muscle pain, and relax the nervous system.

Relaxing Epsom Salts Bath

Unlike the hot bath described in Chapter 9, this is a warm bath and is therefore excellent just before bed. Temperatures that are too hot or too cold can be temporarily stimulating but a warm Epsom salts bath is just right. Epsom salts are a rich source of magnesium, which is absorbed through the skin in the bath and produces deep relaxation of both the nervous and muscular systems. Use this bath as often as desired. It's especially helpful if you are feeling emotionally tense or if you are suffering from muscle pain.

• Make your bath-time tranquil by dimming the lights, lighting a candle, playing your favorite relaxing music, and making sure that no one will disturb you.

• Fill your bathtub with comfortably warm water, adding 2 cups of Epsom salts to the tub while the water is running. Stir the water with your hand to dissolve the salts.

• For additional relaxing benefits, add ten drops of lavender essential oil to the water after the tub has filled, again stirring the water with your hand to disperse the oil (see Aromatherapy on page 116).

• Soak in the water for fifteen to thirty minutes, adding hot water as needed to maintain a comfortably warm temperature.

• Drain the water from the tub and use your imagination to visualize that

any remaining tension is being carried down the drain with the bathwater.

• Gently pat yourself dry and get into bed for a relaxing night's sleep.

Lymph-Stimulating Footbath

Alternating between hot and cold footbaths in one sitting stimulates lymphatic flow and also relieves tired, aching feet and legs. Try this hydrotherapy technique before bed to treat restless legs syndrome and to prevent
nighttime leg cramps. You can use these footbaths as often as desired.

• You'll need two buckets that are each large enough to hold both of your
  feet and ideally deep enough so that the water will reach to the middle
  of your calves.

• Fill one bucket with water as hot as you can tolerate, approximately
  105–110°F. Fill the other bucket with ice-cold water, approximately 55–
  65°F (you may need to add ice cubes to reach the desired temperature).
  Add five drops of rosemary essential oil (see Therapeutic Essential Oils
  on page 117) to the bucket of hot water to further stimulate circulation.

• Sitting in a comfortable chair, immerse both of your feet in the hot
  water for three minutes. Immediately plunge your feet into the bucket of
  cold water for one minute.

• Repeat the hot-to-cold cycle three to five times, ending with the cold-
  water plunge.

AROMATHERAPY

Essential oils give many flowers, herbs, spices, and fruits their characteristic scents. But as ancient peoples knew, the benefits of essential oils go far
beyond their pleasing aromas to the practice of aromatherapy, in which
scents are utilized for their noticeable effects on physical and psychological states. The famed Greek physician Hippocrates had a delightful prescription for longevity: a daily soak in a scented bath, followed by an
aromatherapy massage. Researchers today are confirming his beliefs by
proving that essential oils have measurable effects on both the body and
the emotions. These concentrated plant essences retain the healing properties of the herbs and flowers from which they are distilled and can be
used for treating both physical and psychological disorders.

When essential oils are inhaled or applied to the skin, the aromatic molecules enter the bloodstream and are circulated throughout the body. Oils can be used in this way to address a variety of physical conditions, from fighting respiratory infections to relieving digestive upsets, headaches, premenstrual syndrome (PMS), and insomnia. Essential oils affect the emotions, however, through a different physiological pathway. Scents are detected in the nose by olfactory cells that connect directly with the central nervous system. The olfactory nerve pathways are linked to the limbic portion of the brain, which is the seat of our emotions, memories, intuition, and sexual response. That's why, of all the senses, smell is the most influential trigger of memories and emotions; it's also why aromatherapy can be so helpful for relaxation and stress relief.

Scientific Support for Aromatherapy

Researchers have discovered that smelling the fragrances of various essential oils has distinct effects on brainwave patterns as recorded by a polygraph. Inhaling oils thought to be stimulating (such as black pepper, rosemary, and basil) increase beta waves, which indicate a state of heightened awareness. Oils presumed to be calming (such as neroli, jasmine, lavender, and rose) produce more alpha and theta waves, indicative of relaxation and well-being.

Further experiments have demonstrated that aromatherapy can even be used to promote sleep onset and extend sleep duration. In a study reported in 1996 in the British medical journal *Lancet*, elderly patients suffering from insomnia found that the aroma of lavender helped them to fall asleep more quickly and to sleep longer than did prescription sedatives. A number of other studies have reported similar findings and research continues in the attempt to validate the therapeutic uses of essential oils.

Therapeutic Essential Oils

Some essential oils help relieve tension, anxiety, and depression, and others specifically promote restful sleep. Some, on the other hand, have an energizing effect that's helpful for counteracting the daytime fatigue often associated with insomnia—these stimulating oils, obviously, shouldn't be used at bedtime (for quick reference, see the inset "Aromatherapy at a Glance" on page 121).

On occasion, you may even choose to combine relaxing and stimulating oils, as in the following aromatherapy recommendation for jet lag, which uses lavender to alleviate emotional tension, sandalwood for relaxation, and grapefruit to uplift and energize. Add six drops each of lavender and sandalwood to a warm bath to help you relax before bed; in the morning, place three drops each of lavender and grapefruit oil on a damp washcloth and use it to scrub your body under a warm shower; follow with a cool-water rinse.

This list of essential oils can be consulted for the relief of symptoms of sleep disorders and a number of other conditions.

- Basil alleviates depression and helps restore mental clarity. It relieves headaches, sinus congestion, indigestion, and sore muscles. The sweet, spicy, balsamic fragrance of basil blends well with bergamot, clary sage, rosemary, and peppermint.

- Bergamot has an uplifting quality and eases anxiety and depression. It has antiseptic properties and is helpful for respiratory tract infections and indigestion. The fresh, spicy, citrus-floral scent of bergamot combines well with basil, lavender, orange, and peppermint.

- Chamomile is soothing for both body and mind. It calms anxiety and stress, relieves insomnia, and is excellent for children. It also helps ease headaches, digestive distress, and menstrual cramps. The slightly sweet, herbaceous fragrance of chamomile blends well with geranium, lavender, orange, and patchouli.

- Clary sage is deeply relaxing and has powerful antidepressant properties. It helps ease muscle pain, PMS, and menopausal symptoms. Use this oil in moderation, unless you want a sedative effect. The complex, sweet, herbaceous scent of clary sage combines well with bergamot, lavender, sandalwood, and ylang ylang.

- Cypress relieves emotional stress and insomnia. It increases circulation and is therefore helpful for varicose veins and water retention. The pungent, sweet, balsamic scent of cypress combines well with clary sage, lavender, orange, and sandalwood.

- Geranium helps ease tension and emotional stress and is useful for PMS or menopausal discomfort. The citrus-rose fragrance of geranium blends well with bergamot, lavender, patchouli, and rose.

- Lavender is soothing and relaxing and helps restore physical and emotional well-being. It eases anxiety, tension, fatigue, headaches, and PMS symptoms. The sweet, floral, herbaceous fragrance of lavender combines well with bergamot, clary sage, orange, peppermint, and sandalwood.

- Orange is mood-brightening and creates an overall feeling of well-being. The fresh citrus fragrance of orange combines well with clary sage, lavender, and sandalwood.

- Patchouli is calming and helps relieve stress, emotional fatigue, and insomnia. Good-quality patchouli has a rich earthy fragrance that combines well with clary sage, geranium, lavender, orange, and sandalwood.

- Peppermint is stimulating and energizing and helps allay physical and mental fatigue. It relieves digestive distress and eases tension headaches. The potent, refreshing, menthol scent of peppermint combines well with basil, bergamot, lavender, and rosemary.

- Rose has gentle relaxing properties and helps alleviate nervous tension and associated complaints such as headaches and insomnia. It also eases grief and depression and is considered to be an aphrodisiac. The deep, sweet, floral fragrance of rose blends well with clary sage, lavender, and sandalwood.

- Rosemary is stimulating and counteracts mental and physical fatigue. It increases circulation, eases muscle soreness, and relieves respiratory congestion. The strong, minty, balsamic fragrance of rosemary combines well with basil, lavender, and peppermint.

- Sandalwood, used for centuries as perfume and incense, promotes calmness and serenity. The warm, woody, complex fragrance of sandalwood blends well with bergamot, clary sage, lavender, patchouli, and rose.

- Ylang ylang has strong sedative properties and helps ease depression, frustration, and insomnia. It also has aphrodisiac properties. The intensely sweet, floral fragrance of ylang ylang combines well with bergamot, orange, and sandalwood.

How to Use Essential Oils

The following are a few of the many ways that you can bring the pleasure and benefits of fragrant essential oils into your life, whether as a quick pick-me-up or as a calming, stress-relieving, and sleep-enhancing treatment.

Baths

Add three to ten drops of essential oil to a bathtub of warm water. To prevent possible skin irritation, first dilute the essential oil in 1 teaspoon of vegetable oil or liquid soap. You can also mix ten drops of essential oil with 1 cup of Epsom salts or baking soda in a plastic container, shake well, and then add it to the bathtub, stirring the water to dissolve the mixture. Soaking for ten to twenty minutes in an aromatherapy bath is a good way to experience the benefits of essential oils; the bath can be relaxing or energizing, depending on the oil used.

Massage

Add ten drops of essential oil to 1 ounce of almond, grapeseed, or jojoba oil and use as you would any massage oil. Aromatherapy massage is excellent for deep relaxation, easing muscle stiffness, improving lymphatic circulation, and enhancing overall well-being.

Simple Inhalation

Place one drop of essential oil onto a handkerchief or tissue and inhale as desired. Depending on the oil used, inhalation aromatherapy can alleviate stress, improve concentration, or clear the sinuses.

Room Spray

Add six drops of essential oil to 1 cup of water in a clean spray-bottle. Shake well and use as you would any air freshener. To prevent staining, avoid spraying the mixture onto wood surfaces or upholstered furniture. An aromatherapy air freshener provides a calming or energizing influence, depending on the oil used.

Cautions for Essential Oils

Essential oils are very safe when used appropriately and according to the following precautions.

- In general, do not use undiluted essential oils on your skin without the advice of a professional. Undiluted essential oils can cause skin irritation.

- Do not take essential oils internally without the guidance of a qualified aromatherapy practitioner.

- Keep essential oils away from your eyes.

- Avoid oils that can cause photosensitivity. Bergamot (unless it is labeled as bergapten-free), lemon, lime, and orange essential oils can all cause uneven skin pigmentation if used topically within four hours of exposure to sunlight.

- Keep essential oils out of the reach of children. When using essential oils for children, use only nontoxic and non-irritating oils such as lavender and chamomile.

- Use essential oils with caution during pregnancy. In general, use half of the usual adult dosage while pregnant and stick with non-stimulating oils such as chamomile, lavender, geranium, grapefruit, neroli, rose, and sandalwood.

Aromatherapy at a Glance

Relaxing Essential Oils	Energizing Essential Oils
Chamomile (*Matricaria recutita*)	Basil (*Ocimum basilicum*)
Clary sage (*Salvia sclarea*)	Bergamot (*Citrus bergamia*)
Frankincense (*Boswellia carterii*)	Eucalyptus (*Eucalyptus globulus*)
Geranium (*Pelargonium graveolens*)	Grapefruit (*Citrus x paradisi*)
Jasmine (*Jasminum officinale*)	Lemon (*Citrus limon*)
Lavender (*Lavendula angustifolia*)	Lime (*Citrus aurantifolia*)
Marjoram (*Origanum majorana*)	Orange (*Citrus sinensis*)
Neroli (*Citrus aurantium*)	Peppermint (*Mentha piperita*)
Patchouli (*Pogostemon cablin*)	Rosemary (*Rosmarinus officinalus*)
Rose (*Rosa* spp.)	Sweet orange (*Citrus sinensis*)
Sandalwood (*Santalum album*)	
Ylang ylang (*Cananga odorata*)	

12

Sleep Medications and Why You Should Avoid Them

As you've learned from reading this book, there are a variety of natural approaches to the treatment of sleep disorders, from lifestyle and behavioral therapies to herbs and dietary supplements. But even though numerous studies have demonstrated the effectiveness and safety of herbs and other natural remedies for treating insomnia, many physicians continue to prescribe pharmaceutical sleep-aids, despite the problems of addiction, side effects, and lack of effectiveness over time that these drugs present—and despite the observations of sleep researchers that the sleep induced by a drug is not as restful as normal sleep. In this chapter, you'll learn about different classes of drugs used for sleep problems and why you should avoid taking them.

WHY DOCTORS PRESCRIBE DRUGS

There are several possible reasons that doctors commonly prescribe drugs for treating sleep disorders, rather than suggesting the natural approaches detailed in this book; one reason is the influence of drug manufacturers. Pharmaceutical companies are generally not interested in researching botanical or other natural medicines because of the difficulties in obtaining a patent for an herbal formula. The facts that herbal remedies and nutritional supplements are widely marketed by many independent companies and are available over-the-counter in natural food stores and pharmacies also significantly limit their potential to generate a profit for pharmaceutical manufacturers. Pharmaceutical companies do, however, spend billions of dollars on advertising their drugs, including running ads in the popular media that influence not only what physicians prescribe but also what patients request from their doctors.

Some physicians hesitate to prescribe herbs and dietary supplements because they aren't accustomed to using them; or, they may be uncomfortable when the precise active ingredients in a natural remedy have not been identified. This lack of precision is not unusual with herbal medicines, because, as many herbalists and botanical researchers point out, herbs typically contain a wide array of compounds that act synergistically to create a physiological effect in the body. A complete herb often has greater potential for healing than a single chemical constituent isolated from the plant. For example, although hyperforin has been proposed as the primary active ingredient in St. John's wort that relieves depression, additional compounds in the herb seem to support the action of hyperforin and still others may buffer the active ingredients to prevent side effects. Unfortunately, focusing on only one compound while dismissing the rest as unimportant is a short-sighted view that has plagued the integration of many traditional herbal treatments into modern medicine.

COMMON DRUGS FOR SLEEP PROBLEMS

Using pharmaceutical sleep-aids requires attention to their risks and side effects. One of the most common undesirable outcomes to treatment with these medications is dependency. Dependency on a sleep medication can manifest in a variety of ways: for example, the subsequent inability to sleep without the drug; the need to take increasingly larger amounts of the drug over time to achieve the desired effect (this is also referred to as habituation); and the occurrence of unpleasant physical and psychological withdrawal symptoms when an attempt is made to stop taking the drug. Rebound insomnia, which is an increased sleeplessness caused by discontinuing the use of a drug, is another common side effect of prescription sedatives.

The following are some of the most common drugs taken for sleep difficulties, as well as the problems associated with these medications.

Over-the-Counter Sleep Medications

Most over-the-counter sleep-aids such as Nytol, Sominex, and Tylenol PM contain antihistamines (compounds that relieve the respiratory symptoms of colds and allergies), which do cause drowsiness but are not consistently effective for treating sleep disorders. For many people, these drugs also have significant side effects including morning grogginess, dry mouth, blurred vision, ringing in the ears, heart palpitations, constipation, and nausea. For the elderly, over-the-counter sleep medications can cause nervousness and agitation; instead of awakening refreshed and rested, the patient often experiences the opposite.

Short-Acting Sleeping Pills

These relatively new pharmaceutical sleep-aids include Ambien (zolpidem tartrate) and Sonata (zalepon). They temporarily alter neurotransmitter pathways in the brain and have a sedative, muscle-relaxant effect. On the positive side, short-acting sleeping pills are eliminated from the body within six to eight hours and appear to have a low risk of habituation or rebound insomnia. Problems with dependency and rebound insomnia do occur, however, in certain people or with larger doses. The most commonly reported side effects of these drugs include headache, dizziness, and nausea.

Antidepressants

Because sleep problems are a common symptom of depression, antidepressants are often prescribed to patients whose primary complaint is actually insomnia. Although antidepressants may have a sedative effect and can help regulate the sleep/wake cycle, they also can have a negative effect on REM sleep in particular and sleep quality in general.

Selective serotonin-reuptake inhibitors (SSRIs) such as Prozac are currently the most common drugs for treating depression and are widely prescribed but they are not the benign substances that many doctors believe them to be. Side effects of these drugs include nervousness, fatigue, insomnia, anxiety, gastrointestinal upset, dry mouth, and dizziness. Dependency on SSRIs is common and withdrawal can cause side effects such as dizziness, fatigue, nausea, poor concentration, and irritability.

A disorder called "serotonin syndrome" can occur if too much of an SSRI is taken or if it is combined with other drugs (or with 5-HTP supplements: see Cautions for 5-HTP on page 91) that increase serotonin levels. Symptoms of serotonin syndrome include agitation, confusion, and irregular heartbeat and blood pressure.

Benzodiazepines

Prescribed in small doses as muscle relaxants and for treating anxiety or depression, benzodiazepines such as ativan, Halcion (triazolam), oxazepam, bromazepam, and Valium (diazepam) are also used in larger doses as sleep-aids because of their pronounced sedative effects. Although these drugs are effective in inducing sleep, benzodiazepine abuse and addiction pose a significant problem; dependency can occur in as little as four weeks. The possible side effects of benzodiazepines are numerous and include loss of coordination, confusion, depression, agitation, lethargy, memory impairment, headache, nausea, and heart rhythm disturbances. Many other drugs including alcohol, prescription pain medications, and antihistamines can have dangerous interactions with benzodiazepines and can intensify their effects.

GENERAL CAUTIONS FOR SLEEP MEDICATIONS

It's important to understand that most medications prescribed for a sleep problem are meant for short-term use, with the intention of providing your body the opportunity to resume a normal sleeping pattern that should then sustain itself without further pharmacological assistance. But in reality, many people end up taking these drugs for months or even years. Most pharmaceutical sleep-aids lose their effectiveness with continual use; increasingly higher doses are then required in order to produce a sedative effect. In addition, many are addictive. Stopping the use of a sleep medication often causes rebound insomnia, which then creates the need to resume taking the drug, setting up a cycle of insomnia and drug dependency that is very difficult to break.

If you decide to use a prescription sleep-aid, observe the following cautions.

- Take the drug for no more than a week or two, or no more than once or twice a week over a longer period of time, unless instructed otherwise by your physician (for example, in the case of an SSRI prescribed for narcolepsy or for secondary insomnia associated with depression).

- Whatever pharmaceutical sleep-aid you may use, take the smallest dose that is effective for you. Residual amounts of the drug stay in your body, so your coordination and mental performance are likely to be affected the following day. Taking smaller amounts of the drug will help lessen this effect.

- Never combine sleeping pills with alcohol or any drugs or herbs that have sedative properties. The risks include excessive sedation, headache, rebound insomnia, morning grogginess, respiratory depression (slowed, shallow breathing that lowers blood oxygen levels), and even coma or death.

- Conversely, using any kind of stimulant including caffeine and nicotine will interfere with the effectiveness of a drug treatment taken for a sleep disorder.

CONCLUSION

On the Path to a
Better Night's Sleep

I
n this book, you've learned a great deal about sleep problems: how they arise, the many forms they take, and the situations and conditions that contribute to them. You've also discovered that there are many natural approaches you can take to help your body come back into a balanced state that will allow you to once again enjoy restful sleep.

If you have a sleep problem, you'll most likely need to make some changes in your life to ensure a good night's sleep. By learning to adapt to all of the challenges in your life—positive and negative—so that you are not in distress, you can prevent stress from taking a toll on your physical and emotional well-being. By adopting healthful coping strategies, you can use stress to facilitate your own growth and self-confidence and you can strengthen your ability to handle future stressors. Unlike prescription drugs, which at best will simply sedate you, the suggestions in this book will help you naturally regain the ability to sleep well. At the same time, following the recommendations in this book will improve your overall health and well-being, a positive side effect that prescription drugs can't claim.

You need to keep certain considerations in mind when incorporating natural methods and remedies into your own health care. Many people erroneously believe, for example, that any substance that is naturally derived or is part of a plant cannot be harmful, but the reality is that herbs and supplements have healing benefits because they contain compounds that have measurable biological effects on the body. As with pharmaceuticals, some of these compounds are potentially harmful if used improperly. It's important to realize that herbs and dietary supplements, however, don't fall under the regulation of the U.S. FDA because they are considered to be nutritional supplements rather than drugs. To complicate the issue further, most conventionally trained doctors receive little or no training in nutritional or herbal medicine. Your doctor may not be fully aware of the beneficial properties of herbs and dietary supplements for treating sleep disorders, may not know exactly how to prescribe them, or may be unaware of the precautions that should be observed.

The renaissance of interest in alternative medicine in this country indicates that people are tired of the side effects and costs of prescription medications and are interested in a more natural, less invasive approach to healing. Herbal and nutritional remedies also offer you the opportunity for a more empowered role within your health care, one that enables you to assume a more active role in your healing. This opportunity, however, brings responsibility with it. It is essential to be educated about any substances that you take into your body, whether these substances are prescription drugs, herbs, or dietary supplements. Don't hesitate to seek the help of a healthcare practitioner who is skilled in natural medicine to assist you in your journey. Follow the suggestions in this book and you should be well on your way to consistently restful sleep.

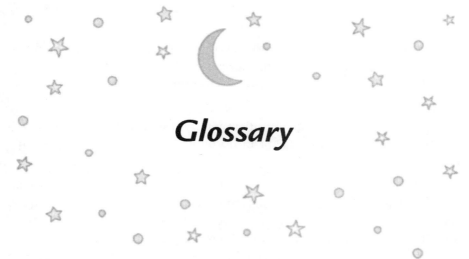

Glossary

Acute insomnia: insomnia that is short-term and temporary; acute insomnia is most often caused by some type of emotional stress or excitement.

Adrenal glands: small glands located on top of the kidneys; the adrenal glands produce hormones that play an important role in the body's response to stress.

Adrenaline: a hormone released by the adrenal glands in response to stressful situations; excessive adrenaline production causes anxiety and insomnia.

Benign prostatic hypertrophy (BPH): the medical term for non-cancerous enlargement of the prostate gland; one of the most common symptoms of BPH is the need to urinate frequently during the night.

Benzodiazepines: a class of prescription drugs (Valium is a well-known example) commonly prescribed to treat anxiety and severe stress; benzodiazepines have numerous side effects and are highly addictive.

Chronic insomnia: insomnia that persists for weeks or months; people with chronic insomnia often suffer from disrupted sleep at least three nights a week; causes of chronic insomnia include underlying physical problems, long-term emotional stress, and environmental or lifestyle factors.

Circadian rhythm: (also referred to as the biological clock) a rhythmic pattern governed by an internal "clock" that regulates hundreds of metabolic and other bodily functions including the sleep/wake cycle.

Cognitive therapy: a psychological treatment that focuses on learning to replace negative attitudes with more realistic, rational thoughts; when used for people suffering from insomnia, cognitive therapy concentrates on changing the thoughts, beliefs, and attitudes that are interfering with healthful sleep patterns.

Cortisol: (also referred to as the stress hormone) a hormone secreted by the adrenal glands in response to stress; excess cortisol is an underlying physiological cause of anxiety, nervousness, and insomnia.

Cytokines: chemical messengers that help regulate immune function and play an important role in the body's inflammatory response; cytokine activity is thought to be a significant factor in fibromyalgia and probably in chronic fatigue syndrome.

Electrolytes: trace minerals (such as sodium, potassium, calcium, and magnesium) that exist in a dissolved state and are critical within the tissues of the body for proper nerve and muscle function; excessive perspiration, diarrhea, and diuretics can all upset the body's electrolyte balance.

Endorphins: natural mood-elevating and pain-relieving compounds produced by the brain; stimuli such as exercise can trigger the release of these "feel-good" chemicals.

5-Hydroxytrytophan (5-HTP): a by-product created when the amino acid tryptophan is broken down in the body to make the brain neurotransmitter serotonin; supplemental 5-HTP is made from the seed of an African plant called griffonia (*Griffonia simplicifolia*).

Gastroesophageal reflux: (also known as heartburn) a condition in which the stomach contents, including digestive acids, back up into the esophagus, causing a burning sensation, coughing, choking, and pain or tightness in the mid-chest area; gastroesophageal reflux is a common cause of sleep disturbances.

Hyperforin: a chemical compound in St. John's wort that is considered to be one of the herb's primary active ingredients.

Hypnagogic state: (also referred to as Stage 1 sleep) the first stage of light non-REM sleep; the hypnagogic state is the transition between wakefulness and sleep.

Hypothalamus: a region of the brain concerned with the circadian timing and other aspects of temperature regulation, sleep/wake cycle, blood pressure, respiration, hunger, and sexual function.

Melatonin: a hormone that plays an important role in regulating the sleep/wake cycle and is produced from serotonin by the pineal gland in response to decreasing light levels.

Neurotransmitter: a molecule used in the body or brain as a chemical messenger to transmit signals between nerve cells or regions of the brain; imbalances of neurotransmitters are thought to contribute to problems including sleep disorders and mood disorders.

Nocturnal leg cramp: a painful muscle spasm in the calf (sometimes also in the thigh or foot) that occurs during the night.

Phytoestrogens: a number of plant compounds with weak estrogenic properties that help balance estrogen levels by attaching to receptor sites in the body that are normally occupied by estrogen.

Pineal gland: a pea-sized structure at the base of the brain that plays an important role in regulating the activity of some hormones, including the secretion of melatonin, in establishing circadian rhythms.

Placebo: an inactive substance or treatment that is administered as though it were active; in clinical studies, a placebo is used as a control measure for comparison to help determine the effectiveness of the drug, herb, or supplement being tested.

Progressive muscle relaxation: a technique that involves systematically tensing and then releasing the muscle groups of the body, creating a deep state of relaxation.

Relaxation therapy: a technique for easing the muscle tension, emotional stress, and anxiety that can interfere with sleep; relaxation therapies include deep-breathing exercises, progressive muscle relaxation, meditation, and gentle stretching exercises.

REM sleep: an active stage of sleep characterized by rapid eye movements (hence the acronym REM); during REM sleep, vivid dreaming takes place, heart rate, blood pressure, respiration, and gastric secretions increase, and memories are thought to be organized and stored in the brain.

Restless legs syndrome (RLS): a sleep disorder characterized by uncomfortable sensations in the legs that are generally worse while sitting, lying down, or resting; in RLS, involuntary jerking and twitching of the legs occurs frequently during sleep.

Seasonal affective disorder (SAD): a depressive disorder associated with the decrease in sunlight during the winter; sleep disturbance is a primary symptom of SAD.

Secondary insomnia: insomnia that is caused by a medical problem (such as chronic pain) or a psychiatric disorder (such as depression or anxiety).

Serotonin: a brain neurotransmitter that acts as a natural tranquilizer; serotonin facilitates communication between nerve cells and has calming and mood-enhancing effects.

Sleep apnea: a sleep disorder characterized by an abnormal breathing pattern of loud snoring with pauses in breathing followed by snorts or gasps; sleep apnea is typically caused by overly relaxed tissues at the back of the throat that obstruct the airway.

Sleep debt: the difference between the hours of sleep that you need and the hours that you're actually getting.

Sleep efficiency number: a quantity calculated as average hours of nightly sleep time divided by average hours nightly spent in bed; the sleep efficiency number, expressed as a percentage, is used in sleep restriction therapy.

Sleep hygiene: a program of basic activities and behaviors that promote good sleep; principles of sleep hygiene include establishing a regular time for sleeping and using the bed only for sleep and sex.

Sleep restriction therapy: a treatment for insomnia that creates mild sleep deprivation by restricting the time spent in bed to make it easier to fall asleep and then gradually lengthens the time spent in bed until a full night of restful sleep is obtained (see also sleep efficiency number).

Standardized extract: an herbal product that is processed in a specific, replicable way and guaranteed to contain a specified amount of the herb's presumed primary active ingredients (see also the Appendix).

Stimulus control therapy: a treatment for insomnia that focuses on breaking negative activity and association patterns related to sleeping; basic principles of stimulus control therapy are associating the bedroom with sleep and eliminating activities that trigger undesired nocturnal wakefulness.

Tryptophan: an essential amino acid, found in many foods, that is a precursor in the synthesis of serotonin.

Choosing and Using Herbs, Nutritional Supplements, and Essential Oils

You've now learned a great deal about the herbs, dietary supplements, and essential oils that can help alleviate sleep problems. Choosing among the vast array of available products, however, can be confusing. In this section, you'll find the information you need to buy, store, and use these natural products with confidence.

BUYING AND STORING HERBS AND SUPPLEMENTS

Walk down the aisle of any natural foods store, supermarket, or drug store and you're likely to find hundreds of nutritional and herbal supplements. When choosing between various brands, you'll probably see a wide variation in price. The more expensive brands are not necessarily better; but as with most things in life, there is usually some correlation between price and quality (in other words, you generally get what you pay for). Another indication of higher-quality products is that they are usually made without artificial colors, preservatives, or sugar.

When it comes to herbal products, there can also be significant differences in quality depending on how the herb was grown, harvested, and processed. Although some products are good sources of the beneficial compounds that make herbs so effective, others may contain little or none of the active ingredients. Because manufacturers want consumers to have confidence in herbal products, the herbal industry is moving toward third-party certification; this means that herbal products would be tested by an independent group (such as the nonprofit U.S. Pharmacopeia or NSF International) to ensure that the products meet certain standards, thereby assuring the consumer of purchasing a high-quality product. For most natural healthcare products and practices, however, third-party certification is still in the developmental stage.

Herbal products are available in many forms and can be used according to your preference. Loose dried herbs such as those sold for tea are relatively inexpensive and making tea is a traditional way of using herbs. When buying dried herbs, choose those that have a vibrant color and strong aroma and flavor. Heat, light, and oxygen destroy the medicinal properties of herbs, so you should store them in a tightly lidded glass jar in a cool, dark, dry place (not in the refrigerator) to maintain their freshness and potency; use them within six months. For sleep problems in particular, preparing a cup of herbal tea can be a relaxing ritual that helps you unwind before bed. This is, however, the most time-consuming method of taking herbal remedies and doesn't extract all the medicinal properties of certain herbs—and some herbs simply don't make a pleasant-tasting tea.

Herb capsules and tablets are convenient to take but these forms are often the least potent because they are so highly processed. The tablets can also be difficult to digest and sometimes pass through the digestive system intact. If you choose to take herb capsules, be sure to buy them from a reputable manufacturer and use them within a couple of months.

Liquid herbal extracts contain a combination of herb-derived compounds, water, and food-grade alcohol. Such extracts offer a broader spectrum of a plant's healing properties than teas do because certain compounds that won't dissolve in water will dissolve in alcohol. (Alcohol-free extracts made with vegetable glycerin are also available but glycerin is not as effective at dissolving some herbal compounds.) Extracts are convenient to take and are highly concentrated; $1/2$ teaspoon of liquid extract is equivalent to approximately 1 cup of herbal tea. Liquid extracts retain their potency for at least three years if stored in a cool, dark place.

Extracts and capsules are both available in standardized form, which indicates that the product is processed to contain a specific amount of what is currently believed to be the herb's primary active ingredient. Standardized extracts were originally created to provide consistent treatments and results for scientific studies, as plants vary in potency according to how they are grown, harvested, and processed. Some batches of herbs might not contain enough of the active compound to be effective; standardization eliminates this problem. Manufacturers use a variety of methods to standardize herbal products, including adding high concentrations of the purified active ingredient and removing what are thought to be unimportant constituents. Many herbalists believe, however, that the other constituents in a whole herb are just as important as the identified (or presumed) active ingredient, including compounds that may provide support for the active ingredient or may help buffer any side effects.

As with herbs, it's important to buy vitamins, minerals, and other nutritional supplements in the form that most appeals to you. Some people have trouble swallowing large tablets. Hard tablets can also be difficult for your body to digest and break down efficiently; capsules of powdered supplements or softgel capsules, however, are usually easier to assimilate. To maintain the potency of your supplements, store them in a cool, dark, dry place such as a kitchen cabinet away from the stove. Don't keep them in the bathroom, because high levels of humidity reduce their potency. Most supplements should not be refrigerated, with the exception of oil-based supplements in bottles or gel capsules (for example, flaxseed oil taken by the spoonful or vitamin E in capsules).

TAKING HERBS AND SUPPLEMENTS

To obtain the maximum benefit from the supplements and herbs that you take, it's helpful to follow a few simple guidelines.

Most supplements are assimilated best when taken with or just after a meal. This is especially true for supplements such as vitamins A, D, and E that are better absorbed with a meal containing some fat. Taking supplements with meals also helps prevent the digestive upset that can occasionally occur if you take them on an empty stomach. Liquid herbal supplements, on the other hand, seem to be best absorbed on an empty stomach. Take them a few minutes before a meal and dilute the dose with a small amount of water or juice to make it more palatable.

It's best to divide supplement dosages so that you're taking them two or three times a day instead of all at once. This provides your body with a continuing supply of nutrients throughout the day, improves absorption, and minimizes the amount that is excreted. It's also best to take nutritional supplements consistently. It often takes a month or two to obtain the full benefits of supplements; for some herbs, it can take three months or even longer, particularly for energy-building herbs such as ashwagandha (*Withania somnifera*) and Siberian ginseng (*Eleutherococcus senticosus*).

Some supplements, particularly herbal products, tend to vary greatly in potency. If you're uncertain about how much you should take, it's safe to follow the manufacturer's recommendations on the label. For general use of an herb, you may wish to try a whole herb extract first and then, if you don't start to see some results after a month, switch to a standardized extract and see whether there is a noticeable difference (remember, though, that it can take three months for the full benefits of an herb or an extract to become apparent). If you are in doubt about what form of an herbal product to use, consult a qualified herbalist for guidance.

BUYING AND STORING ESSENTIAL OILS

Here are a few guidelines to help you select good-quality essential oils and store them correctly.

- Avoid oils labeled as "perfume oil," "fragrance oil," or "nature-identical oil." This indicates that the oil is not a pure essential oil.

- Buy essential oils in dark glass bottles. This protects the oil from the damaging effects of heat and light.

- To best preserve the healing properties of essential oils, store them in a cool, dark place.

- The shelf life of most essential oils is approximately two years (one year for citrus oils). Some oils (sandalwood, frankincense, and patchouli, for example) improve with age.

Selected References

Akhondzadeh S, Naghavi HR, Vazirian M, et al. "Passionflower in the treatment of generalized anxiety: a pilot double-blind randomized controlled trial with oxazepam." *Journal of Clinical Pharmacy and Therapeutics* 2001;26: 363–367.

Connor KM, Davidson JR. "A placebo-controlled study of *Kava kava* in generalized anxiety disorder." *International Clinical Psychopharmacology* 2002;17: 185–188.

Cerny A, Schmid K. "Tolerability and efficacy of valerian/lemon balm in healthy volunteers (a double-blind, placebo-controlled, multicentre study)." *Fitoterapia* 1999;70:221–228.

Dressing H, Riemann D, Low H, et al. "Insomnia: are valerian/balm combinations of equal value to benzodiazepine? [translated from German]" *Therapiewoche* 1992; 42:726–736.

Edwards BJ, Atkinson G, Waterhouse J, et al. "Use of melatonin in recovery from jet-lag following an eastward flight across 10 time-zones." *Ergonomics* 2000;43: 1501–1513.

Garfinkel D, Laudon M, Nof D, et al. "Improvement of sleep quality in elderly people by controlled-release melatonin." *Lancet* 1995;346:541–544.

Garfinkel D, Zisapel N, Wainstein J, et al. "Facilitation of benzodiazepine discontinuation by melatonin: a new clinical approach." *Archives of Internal Medicine* 1999;159:2456–2460.

Gyllenhaal C, Merritt SL, Peterson SD, et al. "Efficacy and safety of herbal stimulants and sedatives in sleep disorders." *Sleep Medicine Reviews* 2000;4: 229–251.

Haimov I, Lavie P, Laudon M, et al. "Melatonin replacement therapy of elderly insomniacs." *Sleep* 1995;18:598–603.

Holzl J, Godau P. "Receptor binding studies with *Valeriana officinalis* on the benzodiazepine receptor." *Planta Medica* 1989;55:642.

Houghton PJ. "The biological activity of Valerian and related plants." *Journal of Ethnopharmacology* 1988;22:121–142.

Hughes RJ, Sack RL, Lewy AJ. "The role of melatonin and circadian phase in age-related sleep-maintenance insomnia: assessment in a clinical trial of melatonin replacement." *Sleep* 1998;21:52–68.

Jussofie A, Schmiz A, Hiemke C. "Kavapyrone-enriched extract from *Piper methysticum* as modulator of the GABA binding site in different regions of rat brain." *Psychopharmacology* 1994;116:469–474.

Kahn RS, Westenberg HG, Verhoeven WM, et al. "Effect of a serotonin precursor and uptake inhibitor in anxiety disorders; a double-blind comparison of 5-hydroxytryptophan, clomipramine and placebo." *International Clinical Psychopharmacology* 1987;2:33–45.

Kennedy DO, Scholey AB, Tildesley NT, et al. "Modulation of mood and cognitive performance following acute administration of *Melissa officinalis* (lemon balm)." *Pharmacology, Biochemistry, and Behavior* 2002;72:953–964.

Larzelere MM, Wiseman P. "Anxiety, depression, and insomnia." *Primary Care* 2002;29:339–360, vii.

Lee KM, Jung JS, Song DK, et al. "Effects of *Humulus lupulus* extract on the central nervous system in mice." *Planta Medica* 1993;59(suppl):A691.

Morin CM, Rodrigue S, Ivers H. "Role of stress, arousal, and coping skills in primary insomnia." *Psychosomatic Medicine* 2003; 65:259–267.

Poldinger W, Calanchini B, Schwarz W. "A functional-dimensional approach to depression: serotonin deficiency as a target syndrome in a comparison of 5-hydroxytryptophan and fluvoxamine." *Psychopathology* 1991;24:53–81.

Soulimani R, Fleurentin J, Mortier F, et al. "Neurotropic action of the hydroalcoholic extract of *Melissa officinalis* in the mouse." *Planta Medica* 1991;57:105–109.

Speroni E, Billi R, Mercati V, et al. "Sedative effects of crude extract of *Passi-flora incarnata* after oral administration." *Phytotherapy Research* 1996;10: S92–S94.

Volz HP, Kieser M. "Kava-kava extract WS 1490 versus placebo in anxiety dis-orders—a randomized placebo-controlled 25-week outpatient trial." *Phar-macopsychiatry* 1997;30:1–5.

Vorbach EU, Gortelmeyer R, Bruning J. "Therapy for insomniacs: effective-ness and tolerance of valerian preparations [translated from German]." *Psychopharmakotherapie* 1996;3:109–115.

Vgontzas AN, Bixler EO, Lin HM, et al. "Chronic insomnia is associated with nyctohemeral activation of the hypothalamic-pituitary-adrenal axis: clinical implications." *Journal of Clinical Endocrinology and Metabolism* 2001;86: 3787–3794.

Yang CM, Spielman AJ, D'Ambrosio P, et al. "A single dose of melatonin pre-vents the phase delay associated with a delayed weekend sleep pattern." *Sleep* 2001; 24:272–281.

Resources

American Academy of Sleep Medicine

6301 Bandel Road, Suite 101
Rochester, MN 55901
507-287-6006
www.asda.org

National Center on Sleep Disorders Research

National Heart, Lung, and Blood Institute, NIH
6705 Rockledge Drive
One Rockledge Centre, Suite 6022
Bethesda, MD 20892-7993
301-435-0199 (phone)
301-480-3451 (fax)

National Sleep Foundation

1522 K Street, NW, Suite 500
Washington, DC 20005
202-347-347
www.sleepfoundation.org

Index

T

U

V

STHE
INATRA
SOLUTION
METABOLIC CARDIOLOGY

Stephen T. Sinatra, M.D., F.A.C.C.

Introduction by James C. Roberts, M.D., F.A.C.C.

Achieve renewed heart health and general well-being with Dr. Sinatra's energy-enhancing nutritional approach.

There's no doubt about it—people with heart disease lack energy. The heart needs a large amount of oxygenated blood flow to continuously meet its huge energy demands. That's where the new triad of cardiac health combination of these energy-supplying nutrients maximizes the amount of oxygen that the heart and skeletal muscle can extract from the blood by accelerating the rate at which cells convert nutrients to energy.

In *The Sinatra Solution*, board-certified cardiologist Dr. Stephen T. Sinatra discusses the importance of energy metabolism on cardiovascular health and the positive impact these three energy-supplying nutrients have on the cardiovascular system. Dr. Sinatra knows that understanding energy metabolism in the heart is critical to devising effective therapies for treating heart disease. He guides readers through the basics of energy metabolism and cardiac bioenergetics, and clearly explains the roles of ribose, carnitine, and CoQ_{10} in the body and specifically how they affect heart health. He provides concise and informative examples of case histories and scientific studies that are testament to the important contribution the supplemental use of these energy-supplying nutrients makes in the lives of people with heart disease every day. This book also touches upon the positive effect the triad has on other diseases and disorders.

About the Author: Stephen T. Sinatra, M.D., F.A.C.C, is a board-certified cardiologist, a certified bioenergetic psychotherapist, and a certified nutrition and antiaging specialist. At his practice in Manchester, Connecticut, Dr. Sinatra integrates conventional medicine with complementary nutritional and psychological therapies to help heal the heart.

Health/Nutrition/Alternative Medicine • Hardcover U.S. $24.95/Can. $39.95 • 240 pages • 6 x 9 • ISBN: 1-59120-158-6

NEW HOPE FOR PREVENTING AND TREATING HEART DISEASE

STHE
INATRA
SOLUTION
METABOLIC CARDIOLOGY*

*me-tab-o-lism (mə -ˈta-bə-li-zəm), n. : the biochemical changes in living cells by which energy is provided for vital processes and activities.

Discover the triad of cardiac health—Coenzyme Q_{10}, L-Carnitine, and D-Ribose. In combination, they help prevent and overcome heart disease, fibromyalgia, chronic fatigue, and Syndrome X.

Stephen T. Sinatra, M.D., F.A.C.C.

Introduction by James C. Roberts, M.D., F.A.C.C.

WAKING THE WARRIOR GODDESS

DR. CHRISTINE HORNER'S PROGRAM TO PROTECT AGAINST & FIGHT BREAST CANCER

Christine Horner, M.D., F.A.C.S.

Harnessing the Power of Nature & Natural Medicines to Achieve Extraordinary Health

DR. CHRISTINE HORNER'S PROGRAM TO
PROTECT AGAINST & FIGHT BREAST CANCER

WAKING THE WARRIOR GODDESS

Harnessing the Power of Nature & Natural
Medicines to Achieve Extraordinary Health

Christine Horner, M.D., F.A.C.S.

Breast cancer has reached epidemic proportions in the United States. Once a relatively rare disease, it now affects 2 to 3 million women, and the incidence is going up at an alarming rate. What can we do about it? Christine Horner, M.D., has the prescription: Take healthy organic foods, add a good dose of certain supplements, get the rest and exercise we need, and avoid those things that are bad for our bodies. We each have a Warrior Goddess in us, and it's time to set her free. A pioneer who pushed through federal and state legislation ensuring that breast reconstruction after a mastectomy would be paid for by insurance companies, Dr. Horner lost her own mother to breast cancer. She decided then that her mother's death would not be in vain. Something good would come from it. This legislation was her first gift to her mother's memory, and this book is another.

Using the metaphor of the Warrior Goddess, this book explains something that Ayurveda describes as our "inner healing intelligence." It also explores the various foods and supplements that can enable women to successfully fight breast cancer and claim the healthy body that should be theirs. Dr. Horner tells readers what to avoid and what to embrace, what will poison the Warrior Goddess and what will feed her and what she needs to thrive.

About the Author: Christine Horner, M.D., F.A.C.S., is a nationally known surgeon, residing in Taos, New Mexico. She holds two board certifications: the National Board of Surgery and the National Board of Plastic Surgery. Dr. Horner was recognized as a leader in her field after she initiated, organized, and managed a successful national campaign to pass laws requiring insurance companies to pay for breast reconstruction following mastectomy. For over a decade, Dr. Horner worked with the American Cancer Society. Dr. Horner is a popular, charismatic speaker and, for the last several years, has spoken extensively on natural health topics and natural approaches to breast cancer prevention. In 1997, Dr. Horner was honored by receiving the YWCA Career Women of Achievement Award.

Health/Alternative Medicine • Hardcover • U.S. $24.95/Can. $39.95 • 320 pages • 6 x 9-inch • ISBN: 1-59120-155-1